AF902798

# Experts' Perspectives on Medical Advances

This book series presents Chinese experts' perspectives on recent developments in clinical medicine. Written by leading Chinese experts in related fields, a wide variety of emerging and hot topics in internal medicine, surgery, oncology, neurosurgery, and ophthalmonology, etc., is covered by the series. Each title in this series covers a disease or a group of diseases, focusing on the basic knowledge, development and the latest research progress of clinical practice. This series is a practical and useful resource for researchers and practitioners in related subjects, as well as for general interest readers.

Xizheng Shan • Entong Wang
Editors

# Interpretation of Vertigo Cases

科学技术文献出版社
SCIENTIFIC AND TECHNICAL DOCUMENTATION PRESS
·北 京·

Springer

*Editors*
Xizheng Shan
Department of Otolaryngology Head and Neck Surgery
Beijing Electric Power Teaching Hospital, Capital Medical University
Beijing, China

Entong Wang
Department of Otolaryngology Head and Neck Surgery
Beijing Electric Power Teaching Hospital, Capital Medical University
Beijing, China

ISSN 2948-1023 ISSN 2948-1031 (electronic)
Experts' Perspectives on Medical Advances
ISBN 978-981-99-6994-4 ISBN 978-981-99-6995-1 (eBook)
https://doi.org/10.1007/978-981-99-6995-1

The translation was done with the help of an artificial intelligence machine translation tool. A subsequent human revision was done primarily in terms of content.

© Scientific and Technical Documentation Press 2023

Jointly published with Scientific and Technical Documentation Press
The print edition is not for sale in China (Mainland). Customers from China (Mainland) please order the print book from: Scientific and Technical Documentation Press.
This work is subject to copyright. All rights are solely and exclusively licensed by the Publisher, whether the whole or part of the material is concerned, specifically the rights of reprinting, reuse of illustrations, recitation, broadcasting, reproduction on microfilms or in any other physical way, and transmission or information storage and retrieval, electronic adaptation, computer software, or by similar or dissimilar methodology now known or hereafter developed.
The use of general descriptive names, registered names, trademarks, service marks, etc. in this publication does not imply, even in the absence of a specific statement, that such names are exempt from the relevant protective laws and regulations and therefore free for general use.
The publishers, the authors, and the editors are safe to assume that the advice and information in this book are believed to be true and accurate at the date of publication. Neither the publishers nor the authors or the editors give a warranty, expressed or implied, with respect to the material contained herein or for any errors or omissions that may have been made. The publishers remain neutral with regard to jurisdictional claims in published maps and institutional affiliations.

This Springer imprint is published by the registered company Springer Nature Singapore Pte Ltd.
The registered company address is: 152 Beach Road, #21-01/04 Gateway East, Singapore 189721, Singapore

Paper in this product is recyclable.

# Editorial Board

**Editor-in-Chief** Shan Xizheng

**Deputy Editor-in-Chief** Wang Entong

**Editorial Board**

Chen Yuanxing, Dai Jing, Fan Chunqiu, Gao Yun, Huang Ligui, Jiang Shujun, Leng Hui, Li Jian, Liu Jinmei, Ma Weiya, Mu Xuetao, Pan Songbin, Shan Xizheng, Shen Xueqiang, Shi Liya, Sun Hanjun, SunQing, Wang Entong, Wang Huibing, Wang Ning, Xing Juanli, Yi Haijin, Yu Xinjun, Zhang Chunlin, Zhang Lei, Zhang Li, Zhang Qinghua, Zheng Kefei

# Preface

Vertigo or dizziness is a common clinical symptom and a type of common disease, which is often difficult to diagnose and has complex and diverse causes. It is not easy to get a clear diagnosis of vertigo and often cannot get timely and accurate treatment, and misdiagnosis and mistreatment often occur, which also brings great burden to patients.

The vestibular system, including the central vestibular system and the peripheral vestibular system, together with the visual and proprioceptive systems, sustains the body's balance function, and when abnormalities in the structure and function of these systems occur, they may lead to symptoms of balance dysfunction such as vertigo, dizziness, and imbalance. Vertigo can usually be divided into vestibular vertigo and non-vestibular vertigo, which in turn can be divided into peripheral vertigo and central vertigo according to the location of their lesions. Although central vertigo is not as common as peripheral vertigo, some central vertigo diseases may not be easily recognized due to atypical clinical manifestations in the early stage, for example, some patients with posterior circulation stroke may present with the so-called isolated vertigo symptoms, and some patients with brain tumors may have only positional vertigo as the main complaint, and thus they are easily misdiagnosed as common peripheral vertigo diseases, and the misdiagnosis and mismanagement of these central vertigo diseases may have serious consequences. Although non-vestibular vertigo is less common, these vertigo disorders are easily overlooked in clinical practice and often fail to receive timely and effective treatment. In addition, multiple vertigo disorders may co-exist in the same patient, which not only increases the difficulty of diagnosis and treatment, but also makes some vertigo disorders easy to be missed or misdiagnosed.

Case reports are an important form of medical literature presentation. Reports of rare or difficult and atypical cases of vertigo help us to gain insight into certain vertigo disorders and improve our diagnosis and treatment of vertigo. In the course of medical practice, our understanding of many diseases starts from case reports, such as Ménière's disease reported and described by French doctor Prosper Ménière in 1861, which led to a new understanding of this disease and a gradual improvement of the diagnosis and treatment level of this disease. Therefore, we have organized the relevant experts to compile the book *Interpretation of Vertigo Cases*, including 35 cases of vertigo that are rare, difficult, and characteristic clinical cases, and we hope that readers can learn from these case reports and gain some benefits.

Beijing, China
October 20, 2022

Xizheng Shan

# Contents

# Contributors

**Yuanxing Chen** Institute of Vertigo, Third Medical Center, PLA General Hospital, Beijing, China

**Jing Dai** Institute of Vertigo, Third Medical Center, PLA General Hospital, Beijing, China

**Chunqiu Fan** Department of Neurology, Xuanwu Hospital, Capital Medical University, Beijing, China

**Yun Gao** Institute of Vertigo, Third Medical Center, PLA General Hospital, Beijing, China

**Ligui Huang** Department of Otolaryngology, Head and Neck Surgery, The 908th Hospital of Joint Logistics Support Force of PLA, Nanchang, China

**Shujun Jiang** Department of Comprehensive Treatment, Second Medical Center, Chinese PLA General Hospital, Beijing, China

**Hui Leng** Department of Otolaryngology, Affiliated Hospital of Liaoning Traditional Chinese Medicine University, Shenyang, China

**Jian Li** Institute of Vertigo, Third Medical Center, PLA General Hospital, Beijing, China

**Jinmei Liu** Institute of Vertigo, Third Medical Center, PLA General Hospital, Beijing, China

**Weiya Ma** Department of Neurology, Third Medical Center, PLA General Hospital, Beijing, China

**Xuetao Mu** Department of Magnetic Resonance Imaging, Third Medical Center, PLA General Hospital, Beijing, China

**Songbin Pan** Department of Neurology, Wuhan First Hospital, Wuhan, China

**Xizheng Shan** Institute of Vertigo, Electric Power Teaching Hospital, Capital Medical University, Beijing, China

**Xueqiang Shen** Institute of Vertigo, Third Medical Center, PLA General Hospital, Beijing, China

**Liya Shi** Institute of Vertigo, Electric Power Teaching Hospital, Capital Medical University, Beijing, China

**Hanjun Sun** Department of Otolaryngology, Head and Neck Surgery, Third Medical Center, PLA General Hospital, Beijing, China

**Qing Sun** Institute of Vertigo, Third Medical Center, PLA General Hospital, Beijing, China

**Entong Wang** Institute of Vertigo, Electric Power Teaching Hospital, Capital Medical University, Beijing, China

**Huibing Wang** Department of Otolaryngology, Head and Neck Surgery, Third Medical Center, PLA General Hospital, Beijing, China

**Ning Wang** Institute of Vertigo, Electric Power Teaching Hospital, Capital Medical University, Beijing, China

**Juanli Xing** Department of Otolaryngology, Head and Neck Surgery, First Affiliated Hospital, School of Medicine, Xi'an Jiaotong University, Xi'an, China

**Haijin Yi** Department of Otolaryngology, Head and Neck Surgery, Beijing Tsinghua Changgung Hospital, Tsinghua University, Beijing, China

**Xinjun Yu** Department of Vertigo Medicine, Affiliated Hospital of Weifang Medical College, Weifang, China

**Chunlin Zhang** Department of Neurology, Central Hospital of Liuzhou Railway, Liuzhou, China

**Lei Zhang** Head and Neck Rehabilitation Center, Beijing Rehabilitation Hospital, Capital Medical University, Beijing, China

**Li Zhang** Department of Otolaryngology, Head and Neck Surgery, Affiliated Hospital of Inner Mongolia Medical University, Hohhot, China

**Qinghua Zhang** Institute of Vertigo, Third Medical Center, PLA General Hospital, Beijing, China

**Kefei Zheng** Institute of Vertigo, Third Medical Center, PLA General Hospital, Beijing, China

# Part I

# Peripheral Vertigo Disorders

# Benign Paroxysmal Positional Vertigo Secondary to Laparoscopic Cholecystectomy

1

Ligui Huang and Entong Wang

## 1.1 Summary of Medical Records

Patient, male, 51 years old. Complaint: Five days after laparoscopic cholecystectomy and 1 day of recurrent episodes of vertigo. Present history: The patient was diagnosed with gallstones and cholecystitis due to recurrent episodes of right upper abdominal pain for more than 1 year and was hospitalized in the Department of Hepatobiliary Surgery on May 26, 2015 to undergo laparoscopic cholecystectomy under general anesthesia, which lasted 75 min, and the surgery and postoperative recovery process were relatively smooth; he was discharged 4 days after surgery. However, on the day after discharge, the patient had a sudden onset of vertigo while lying down in bed with a pronounced spinning sensation. The vertigo lasted for a short time, about 10 s, with no specific symptoms other than nausea. Past history: no history of ear disease, no history of hypertension, coronary artery disease, or diabetes mellitus. The patient was then seen at the ENT clinic. Examination: no neurological signs, no abnormal findings on general otologic examination, and no spontaneous nystagmus. The patient was initially considered to be suffering from benign paroxysmal positional vertigo (BPPV). The patient underwent an instrument-assisted positional test with the SRM-IV diagnosis and therapy system for BPPV: the right Dix-Hallpike test was positive, showing a typical vertical torsional nystagmus (Fig. 1.1a, b) with an upward (frontal) vertical component of the nystagmus and a groundward twist of the superior pole of the eye, with a nystagmus latency of 4 s and a duration of 8 s; the roll test was negative. The patient was diagnosed with right posterior semicircular canal BPPV canaloliths. The patient was subsequently treated with canalith repositioning procedure mimicking the Epley maneuver via the SRM-IV diagnosis and therapy system for BPPV. The following day, the patient still presented with episodic vertigo symptom, which occurred mainly when turning in bed. The positional tests were given again, and the Dix-Hallpike test was negative bilaterally, while the roll test was positive, showing geotropic direction-changing horizontal nystagmus (Fig. 1.1c–e), with a nystagmus latency of 4 s, duration of 12 s, and maximum slow-phase velocity of 8.3°/s on the left roll test; the nystagmus latency of 4 s, duration of 20 s, and maximum slow-phase velocity of 20.8°/s on the right roll test. The patient was diagnosed with right horizontal semicircular canal BPPV canaloliths, which was thought to be the result of a "canal

L. Huang
Department of Otolaryngology, Head and Neck Surgery, The 908th Hospital of Joint Logistics Support Force of PLA, Nanchang, China

E. Wang (✉)
Department of Otolaryngology Head and Neck Surgery, Beijing Electric Power Teaching Hospital, Capital Medical University, Beijing, China

© Scientific and Technical Documentation Press 2023

X. Shan, E. Wang (eds.), *Interpretation of Vertigo Cases*, Experts' Perspectives on Medical Advances, https://doi.org/10.1007/978-981-99-6995-1_1

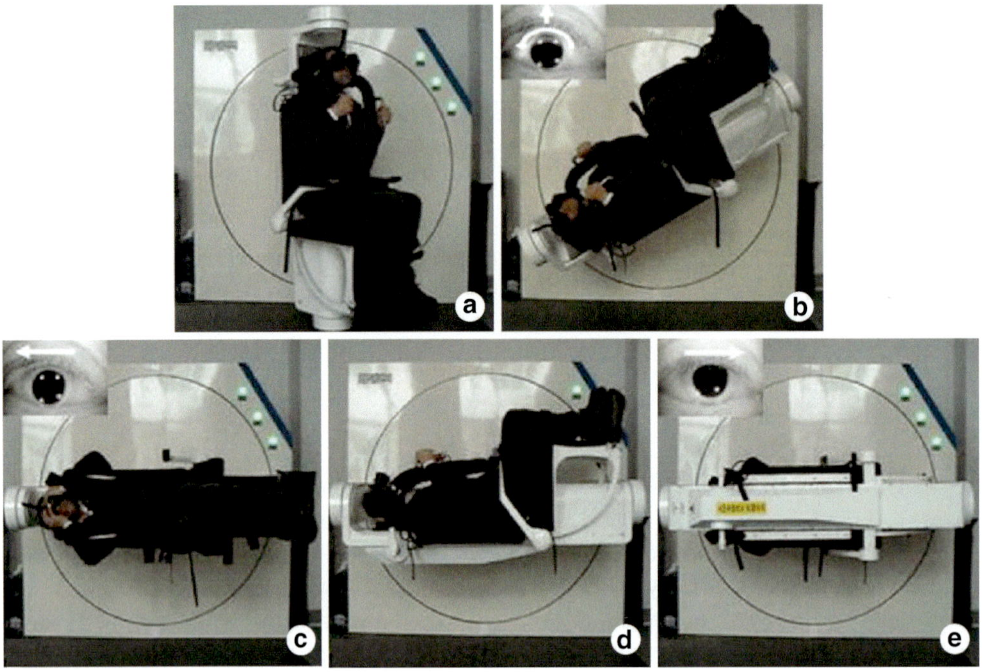

**Fig. 1.1** Schematic diagram of the instrument-assisted diagnostic test. The right Dix-Hallpike test: the patient in upright sitting position with the head turning 45° to the left (**a**) is moved to head-hanging position (**b**), a vertical upbeating nystagmus with counterclockwise torsional component toward the dependent ear is induced, and the nystagmus lasted for 8 s, indicating a diagnosis of right posterior canal BPPV; the roll test: the patient is rolled to the right (**c**) from the neutral position (**d**), inducing geotropic horizontal nystagmus toward the right, and then he is rolled to the left (**e**), provoking weaker geotropic horizontal nystagmus toward the left, suggesting a diagnosis of right horizontal canal BPPV. Arrows depict the directions of nystagmus

switch" after the first canalith repositioning procedure. Five days later, the patient continued to have similar episodes of positional vertigo and the roll test was still positive, so he was re-treated with the barbecue repositioning maneuver. Thereafter, the patient's vertigo symptom was completely resolved and the roll test was negative, and the BPPV was cured. At 1 year and 6 months of follow-up, the patient did not experience any recurrence of BPPV.

## 1.2 Case Study

The patient was a middle-aged male who underwent laparoscopic cholecystectomy under general anesthesia for gallstone cholecystitis and developed recurrent episodes of vertigo induced by head position changes on the fifth postoperative day. The patient had typical symptoms of BPPV, a positive Dix-Hallpike test on the right side and negative on other positional tests, so the initial diagnosis was right posterior semicircular canal BPPV canalolithiasis. The patient was treated with instrument-assisted Epley repositioning maneuver, but after treatment, he continued to exhibit episodes of vertigo with different characteristics from previous vertigo episodes. Upon re-evaluation, the Dix-Hallpike test was negative bilaterally, while the roll test was positive, and the diagnosis of right horizontal semicircular canal BPPV canaloliths was made based on the nystagmus characteristics. At this point, the Dix-Hallpike test turned negative, indicating that the previous right posterior semicircular canal BPPV canalolithiasis had been cured. Since the previous BPPV did not involve the horizontal semicircular canals, this right horizontal semicircular canal BPPV canalolithiasis was probably the result of "canal switch" during the previous canalith repositioning maneuver. In this case, the new emerging BPPV resulting from the "canal switch" was cured after two corresponding repositioning maneuvers. The incidence of "canal switch" is a complication of BPPV treatment, with a frequency of 3% to 6%, and physicians need to be aware of this phenomenon and be able to treat it appropriately. This is a rare case of BPPV secondary to laparoscopic cholecystectomy under general anesthesia and has not been reported to date. The patient's BPPV did not occur immediately after surgery, but only on the fifth postoperative day. The patient had no other concomitant diseases except for a history of gallstones and cholecystitis for more than 1 year, and the surgery was minimally invasive, and the operative time was not long and the bleeding was not much, and the surgical procedure and postoperative recovery were smooth. The patient was followed up for 1 year and 6 months without recurrence of BPPV, and the prognosis was good.

## 1.3 Case Review

BPPV is a common peripheral vestibular disorder and the most common cause of vertigo, which can account for about 30% of vertigo cases. The disease is characterized by brief episodes of vertigo with nystagmus induced by specific head position changes. The etiology and mechanism of BPPV are not yet quite clear. Most cases have an unknown cause and are referred to as primary or idiopathic BPPV, while some cases have a clear or probable cause and are referred to as secondary BPPV. These otolith particles may move within the semicircular canal with the flow of lymphatic fluid (canalolithiasis) or adhere to the cupula. When the head position changes, the vestibular receptors can be stimulated by the action of these otolith particles and vertigo symptoms and nystagmus can be induced. In recent years, BPPV secondary to various surgical procedures has been reported, suggesting that this secondary BPPV is not a very uncommon surgical complication. Because some clinicians do not know enough about this secondary BPPV, it has not been diagnosed and treated in a timely and effective manner, so it needs to be brought to the attention of clinicians and managed appropriately. The occurrence of postoperative secondary BPPV is closely related to the surgical site, intraoperative technique and the patient's body (head) position. BPPV can also occur rarely in non-craniofacial surgeries, such as cardiac and abdominal surgeries and even minimally invasive laparoscopic surgeries. The postoperative secondary BPPV is not significantly related with age and sex, and may be related to the surgical population. The semicircular canals and lateralities involved in postoperative secondary BPPV are related to factors such as surgical site, modality, operating technique, and intraoperative patient's position.

The underlying mechanisms of postoperative secondary BPPV are not well understood and may include the following: (1) Direct injury: mostly seen in ear surgery, where otoliths are dislodged due to damage to the utricle macula. (2) External forces: certain surgical manipulation techniques are also an important factor in the development of BPPV. In otologic, dental, and other craniofacial surgeries involving the temporal bone, jaws, and other cranial bones, instruments such as hammers, chisels, saws, and drills are commonly used to tap and grind the bony structures adjacent to the vestibular organs, and the resulting vibratory effects, especially the percussive forces, may lead to the dislodgement of the otolith of the utricle macula. (3) Influence of surgical position: the position of the patient during surgery may also be a factor in the development of postoperative BPPV. In some surgical procedures, the patient is required to remain in a certain position for a long time during surgery, which may provide an opportunity for a dislodged otolith to enter the semicircular canal, increasing the risk of BPPV. (4) Impaired blood supply to the inner ear: ischemia in the inner ear is also a possible cause for the development of BPPV. Intraoperatively controlled hypotension techniques were commonly used in some surgeries for the reason of surgery itself or the need for anesthesia, which can result in short-term hypotension and hypoperfusion of the inner ear, which may also be associated with the development of secondary BPPV in its postoperative period.

The diagnosis of postoperative secondary BPPV is not very difficult based on its typical symptoms and specific diagnostic positional tests and the corresponding surgical history. Although BPPV is self-limiting and some patients can heal spontaneously with a good prognosis, some patients have a serious impact on their function, activity, and quality of life due to the persistence of BPPV, so its timely treatment is of positive significance. Manual or instrument-assisted repositioning maneuver is an effective treatment for BPPV and has good therapeutic results. However, in the early postoperative period, it is difficult for patients to undergo diagnostic tests and repositioning maneuvers because of their limited physical activity, which makes the diagnosis and repositioning treatment of secondary BPPV after surgery somewhat difficult. If the patient is not able to receive repositioning treatment in the short term due to limited physical activity, he/she may also choose to observe and follow up, waiting for resolving spontaneously, or later the patient may receive repositioning treatment when their physical condition permits. Instrument-assisted diagnostic tests and repositioning maneuvers provide the possibility of timely treatment for such patients, which usually leads to better results and a good prognosis.

## Bibliography

Shan X, Wang A, Wang E. Benign paroxysmal positional vertigo secondary to laparoscopic surgery. Sage Open Med Case Rep. 2017;5:1–4.

Wang E. Benign paroxysmal positional vertigo and its treatment strategies. Beijing Med. 2017;39(8):760–3.

Wang A, Wang E. Benign paroxysmal positional vertigo due to spinal surgery: a case report. J Ear Nose Throat Disord. 2016;1:1005.

Wang E, Shan X, Tan Z. Benign paroxysmal positional vertigo: a not uncommon surgical complication. Chin J Otolaryngol Head Neck Surg. 2015;50(9):787–9.

# Benign Paroxysmal Positional Vertigo Secondary to Hunt Syndrome

2

Songbin Pan

## 2.1 Summary of Medical Records

Patient, female, 61 years old. Complaint: Recurrent episodes of vertigo for 10 days. Present history: In the past 10 days, the patient had recurrent episodes of vertigo, rotating vision, unstable standing and walking, accompanied by nausea and vomiting, without headache and photophobia and phonophobia. She was treated with vasodilators, betahistine, and flunarizine, and the frequency of vertigo attacks decreased; the patient was admitted to the hospital for further diagnosis and treatment. Past history: 2 months before admission, the patient had been hospitalized under the ENT department with herpes zoster in the right ear. While in hospital, she developed vertigo, unstable walking, and hearing loss in the right ear. The patient was later transferred to the Acupuncture Department of our hospital for treatment. During her hospitalization, she developed right-sided facial paralysis that was diagnosed as Hunt syndrome. The patient was given medical treatment with acyclovir, dibazol, prednisone, vitamin B1, methylcobalamin, and so on. The patient had a sudden hearing loss in the left ear with vertigo attacks 10 years ago, which was diagnosed as "Meniere disease." On admission, the patient had no spontaneous nystagmus, positive for head impulse test on the right, Fukuda test with turning to the right, negative Romberg's sign, Romberg's reinforcement test showing unstable and tilting in an indeterminate direction. Right Dix-Hallpike test was positive, inducing vertical rotational nystagmus, i.e., nystagmus vertically upward with counterclockwise rotation of the upper pole of the eye, left Dix-Hallpike test and roll test were negative. On admission, magnetic resonance imaging showed multiple lacunar cerebral infarcts and ischemic foci in the bilateral basal ganglia and centrum semiovale, bilateral frontal lobes, and deep cerebral white matter ischemia; cranial enhancement scan did not show any significant abnormal strengthening foci; bilateral inner ear water imaging did not show any significant abnormal changes. Pure tone hearing threshold measurement: sensorineural deafness in the high frequency region of both ears, with significant hearing loss in the left ear. Caloric test showed mild paralysis of the left horizontal semicircular canal, with a CP value of 58.3%. The patient was diagnosed with benign paroxysmal positional vertigo (BPPV) based on recurrent episodes of positional vertigo over the past 10 days and a positive Dix-Hallpike test on the right side, and was treated with Epley's repositioning maneuver. After 7 days of hospitalization, the patient did not have any further attack of positional vertigo, and the Dix-Hallpike tests and roll tests were negative bilaterally. However, the patient still felt dizzy or unsteadiness when

S. Pan (✉)
Department of Neurology, Wuhan First Hospital, Wuhan, China

© Scientific and Technical Documentation Press 2023
X. Shan, E. Wang (eds.), *Interpretation of Vertigo Cases*, Experts' Perspectives on Medical Advances, https://doi.org/10.1007/978-981-99-6995-1_2

moving too fast or turning around, and the impulse head test was positive on the right side, the Fukuda test showed the patient turned to the right, the Romberg sign was negative, and the Romberg strengthening test showed patient was unstable with uncertain direction of tilting. The patient's poor motion tolerance was considered to be due to residual dysfunction of the vestibular nerve after herpes virus infection and inadequate compensation of vestibular function, and the patient was instructed to continue home vestibular rehabilitation training after discharge. At the follow-up visit 6 weeks after discharge, the patient's vertigo symptoms disappeared and she walked steadily, but her hearing did not change, and the patient occasionally had tinnitus.

## 2.2 Case Study

The patient complained of recurrent vertigo induced by head position change in the last 10 days, her symptoms were consistent with paroxysmal positional vertigo; the right Dix-Hallpike test was positive, and thus she was diagnosed with right posterior semicircular canal BPPV. The patient's vertigo symptoms were significantly relieved after repositioning treatment with the Epley maneuver; no further vertigo symptoms occurred afterwards, and the patient was rechecked after 7 days of hospitalization, showing negative for the bilateral Dix-Hallpike tests and roll test. The patient's good response to the repositioning treatment also supported the diagnosis of BPPV. The patient had a history of herpes zoster virus infection and Hunt syndrome with vertigo for more than 2 months, which was considered to be the result of herpes virus infection involving the right vestibular nerve and labyrinth. The patient's hearing loss on the left side was probably the sequelae of sudden hearing loss in the left ear 10 years ago, but considering that the patient's sudden hearing loss did not have fluctuating changes 10 years ago, and her vertigo symptoms did not show recurrent episodes, it was thought that the disease was probably "sudden deafness with vertigo" rather than "Meniere disease." The mild paralysis of the left semicircular canal, indicated by the caloric test, may be due to the residual vestibular lesion. The patient was discharged from the hospital with poor motion tolerance and balance dysfunction, which was considered to be the result of vestibular neuritis caused by the herpes virus infection. The patient was followed up at 6 weeks after discharge, and the patient's symptoms of balance dysfunction had largely disappeared.

## 2.3 Case Review

This case presented with typical positional vertigo symptoms and a positive Dix-Hallpike test on one side, and was diagnosed with right posterior semicircular canal BPPV after excluding central positional vertigo. According to the current criteria for the diagnosis of BPPV, the complete diagnosis of BPPV should also include the underlying pathophysiological mechanism. The patient's vertigo, provoked by head position change, lasted only a few seconds, and thus, her BPPV should be of the (canalolithiasis) of the right posterior canal. The patient's vertigo symptoms resolved with repositioning treatment, and the Dix-Hallpike test turned negative, indicating that the patient's BPPV diagnosis and repositioning treatment were appropriate. Most cases of BPPV have an unknown etiology and are referred to as idiopathic or primary BPPV. Some cases of BPPV have a definite or probable etiology and are referred to as secondary BPPV, and some of them can be secondary to inner ear vestibular disorders such as Meniere disease, vestibular neuritis, and sudden deafness, but BPPV secondary to Hunt syndrome is relatively rare. Hunt syndrome, also known as geniculate ganglionitis A group of cases with specific symptoms caused by herpes virus infection of the geniculate ganglion of the facial nerve, was first reported by Ramsay Hunt in 1907 and was later referred to as Hunt syndrome or herpes zoster oticus. The syndrome can be clinically classified into three types based on its clinical manifestations: type I, which presents only with ear herpes and otalgia; type II, which, in addition to ear herpes, presents with peripheral facial palsy due to invasion of the facial nerve;

type III, which, in addition to ear herpes and peripheral facial palsy symptoms, can involve the auditory nerve and cause auditory symptoms such as sensorineural hypoacusis, tinnitus, and auditory hypersensitivity, and can also involve the vestibular nerve and labyrinth and cause vestibular symptoms, which can be manifested as episodic vertigo, balance disorder, or unstable walking. In this case, the patient presented as the type III of Hunt syndrome, which was followed by BPPV due to viral infection and inflammatory damage to the vestibule of the inner ear, resulting in the dislodgement of the otolith in the utricle macula. Therefore, in patients with Hunt syndrome who present with vertigo, especially positional vertigo, attention should be paid to the recognition and treatment of secondary BPPV. Some patients with Hunt syndrome have a poor prognosis and may have residual symptoms of facial palsy, hearing loss, and balance dysfunction due to viral damage to the facial and cochleovestibular nerves. This secondary BPPV is easily cured with repositioning maneuver, but balance dysfunction symptoms mostly require a period of vestibular rehabilitation exercises. In addition to the acute treatment of vertigo due to otitis caused by herpes zoster infection, vestibular rehabilitation exercises during the recovery period are equally important. In addition to the hearing loss in the right ear due to this disease, the patient in this case had severe deafness left after sudden hearing loss in the left ear 10 years ago. If the patient's hearing impairment affects her ability to perform daily activities, the patient's hearing rehabilitation should be considered, for example, with the fitting of hearing aids.

## Bibliography

Martin-Sanz E, Rueda A, Esteban-Sanchez J, et al. Vestibular restoration and adaptation in vestibular neuritis and Ramsay Hunt syndrome with vertigo. Otol Neurotol. 2017;38(7):e203–8.

von Brevern M, Bertholon P, Brandt T, et al. Benign paroxysmal positional vertigo: diagnostic criteria. J Vestib Res. 2015;25(3–4):105–17.

# 3 Multiple Sclerosis Combined with Benign Paroxysmal Positional Vertigo

Xinjun Yu and Weiya Ma

## 3.1 Summary of Medical Records

Patient: female, 54 years old. Complaint: Recurrent vertigo attacks and weakness of extremities for 3 months. Present history: The patient began to have recurrent episodes of vertigo with no apparent cause 3 months ago, with rotating vision, accompanied by nausea and vomiting. The vertigo episodes were mostly related to changes in body position, often occurring when getting up or lying in bed, and when turning from side to side in bed. At the same time, in the past 3 months, the patient felt weakness in all limbs, which gradually worsened. She had been treated in a hospital in Shanxi province, and the brain MRI examination reported "multiple ischemic foci in the frontoparietal subcortex and white matter," and the clinical diagnosis was "cerebral infarction." She was diagnosed as "benign paroxysmal positional vertigo" in a hospital in Beijing, and was treated with manual repositioning maneuver, but the vertigo symptoms improved slightly, without significant treatment efficacy. Subsequently, she came to our vertigo clinic. Physical examination: general examination and neurological examination showed no significant abnormalities. Otologic examination: no abnormalities in the external auditory canals and tympanic membranes. Positional test: The SRM-IV diagnostic and treatment system for vertigo was used to perform the positional tests, and the left Dix-Hallpike test was positive, and the right test and the roll test were negative. The diagnosis was "benign paroxysmal positional vertigo of the left posterior semicircular canal." The patient was treated with the SRM-IV diagnostic and treatment system for vertigo using the 360° backward rotation maneuver of the left posterior semicircular canal. After three repositioning maneuvers, the patient's vertigo symptoms improved, and the positional test was negative for the bilateral Dix-Hallpike tests and roll test. A neurology consultation was held, and a brain MRI was recommended to rule out a central lesion. Brain MRI showed multiple scattered oval plaques visible perpendicular to the lateral ventricles (Fig. 3.1), and a preliminary diagnosis of demyelinating disease (multiple sclerosis) was made and further investigations were performed. Biochemical examination of cerebrospinal fluid was taken by lumbar puncture: increased IgG-24 level. Somatosensory evoked potential test of both upper limbs: prolonged N20 latency. The patient was then diagnosed with demyelinating disease, given methylprednisolone shock therapy, and discharged with improvement of symptoms after systemic treatment.

X. Yu
Department of Vertigo Medicine, Affiliated Hospital of Weifang Medical College, Weifang, China

W. Ma (✉)
Institute of Vertigo, Third Medical Center, PLA General Hospital, Beijing, China

© Scientific and Technical Documentation Press 2023
X. Shan, E. Wang (eds.), *Interpretation of Vertigo Cases*, Experts' Perspectives on Medical Advances, https://doi.org/10.1007/978-981-99-6995-1_3

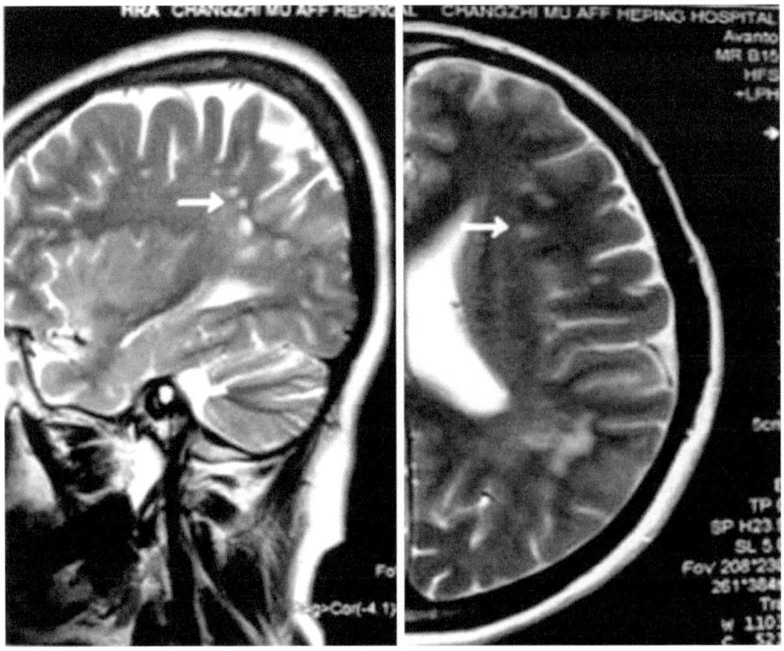


**Fig. 3.1** Brain MRI. Multiple scattered oval plaques (arrows) are seen next to the lateral ventricles

## 3.2 Case Study

The patient was a middle-aged female who complained of recurrent vertigo attacks and weakness of the limbs for 3 months. In a local hospital, the patient was diagnosed with "cerebral infarction" and given medication to improve cerebral blood circulation, but the clinical symptoms did not improve significantly. In another hospital, the patient was diagnosed as "benign paroxysmal positional vertigo" and was treated with manual repositioning maneuver and the vertigo symptoms improved slightly, but the efficacy of treatment was not obvious. The general examination and neurological examination did not reveal any abnormal signs in our vertigo clinic. The patient was diagnosed with "benign paroxysmal positional vertigo of the left posterior semicircular canal" based on a positive Dix-Hallpike test on the left side, a negative test on the right side, and a negative roll test. After the patient was treated with the SRM-IV diagnostic and treatment system for vertigo using the 360° backward rotation maneuver of the left posterior semicircular canal, and three repositioning maneuvers, her vertigo symptoms improved, and the following bilateral Dix-Hallpike tests and roll test were negative, but the patient still had persistent symptoms such as dizziness and weakness of the limbs. The patient had no risk factors for cardiovascular disease and lacked typical symptoms and signs of cerebral infarction, so the reasons for the diagnosis of cerebral infarction was insufficient. After consultation with the neurologist and a brain MRI examination, the patient was found to have multiple scattered oval plaques perpendicular to the lateral ventricles, and she was considered to have "demyelinating disease (multiple sclerosis)." Following somatosensory evoked potential testing of both upper extremities showed prolonged N20 latency. The patient was finally diagnosed with "demyelinating disease (multiple sclerosis)" according to McDonald's diagnostic criteria for multiple sclerosis. After methylprednisolone shock therapy and systemic treatment, the patient's symptoms of dizziness and limb weakness improved, and she was discharged after her symptoms were controlled and was followed up.

## 3.3 Case Review

Benign paroxysmal positional vertigo is the most common cause of vertigo, accounting for about 30% of vertigo cases. It is easy to diagnose benign paroxysmal positional vertigo by repositional test, and the first choice of treatment is particle repositioning maneuver, which is also the most effective treatment for benign paroxysmal positional vertigo, either by manual or instrument-assisted repositioning maneuver. In this case, the diagnosis of benign paroxysmal positional vertigo was clear and the treatment was timely and effective, but the patient still had some symptoms such as dizziness and weakness of the limbs after the benign paroxysmal positional vertigo was cured, suggesting that the patient might have other diseases. Thus the patient was diagnosed with multiple sclerosis and treated accordingly. Some reports in the literature suggest that vertigo attacks in multiple sclerosis can also be caused by concurrent benign paroxysmal positional vertigo.

Demyelinating diseases are a group of diseases whose etiology is not fully understood, in which the lesions occur mainly in the nerve myelin sheath with few changes in the nerve cells themselves. Pathological changes in the acute phase are demyelination, myelin swelling, rupture and inflammation of the tissue. The pathology is characterized by destruction of the myelin sheath of nerve fibers, accompanied by a relative reduction in nerve cells and axons. The pathogenesis is thought to be due to a pathological-immune response in the nervous system. The most common primary demyelinating disease is multiple sclerosis, the pathogenesis of multiple sclerosis is unknown and may be related to a variety of factors, including viral infection, abnormal autoimmune response, genetics, environment, and socioeconomics. Multiple sclerosis is currently considered to be a chronic immune-mediated disease of the central nervous system, and this disease occurs in people aged 10 to 50 years, with more women than men. The lesions can involve the cerebral hemispheres, optic nerve, spinal cord, brainstem, and cerebellum, with clinical symptoms depending on the location of the lesion. The vestibular nucleus and the roots of VIII cranial nerves are common sites of demyelinating lesions, and these lesions can induce vertigo symptoms in patients with multiple sclerosis. Literature reports that among patients with multiple sclerosis, their initial symptoms may be limb weakness (68%), sensory disturbance (43%), visual disturbance (33%), and 20% of patients present with vertigo. The tests and examinations of cerebrospinal fluid cytology and biochemistry, electroencephalography, brain imaging, and so on may be applied to patients with multiple sclerosis. Cerebrospinal fluid biochemistry often shows significant increases in cell count, protein level, and IgG level, and also increased myelin basic protein in the active phase. EEG may show abnormal slowing activity. Evoked potentials can indicate the presence of impaired conduction pathways. Brain MRI often shows multiple scattered plaques that can occur anywhere in the white matter of the brain, but are more common in the brainstem, the cerebellum, and periventricular sites, with plaques that often are oval in shape and perpendicular to the long axis of the lateral ventricles. Demyelinating disease is mainly treated with hormonal therapy, additional treatments include cranial pressure reduction, supportive therapy, symptomatic treatment during attacks, physiotherapy rehabilitation, and psychosocial treatment. Due to the advances in therapeutics, generally the patient can survive for more than 30 years. The case we present suggest that the diagnosis and treatment of vertigo must be meticulous and comprehensive, and that the other possible causes of vertigo should be considered when the clinical manifestations of the patient cannot be explained by single vertiginous disorder.

## Bibliography

Eskandarieh S, Heydarpour P, Minagar A, et al. Multiple sclerosis epidemiology in East Asia, South East Asia and South Asia: a systematic review. Neuroepidemiology. 2016;46(3):209–21.

Perry M, Swain S, Kemmis-Betty S, et al. Multiple sclerosis: summary of NICE guidance. BMJ. 2014;349:g5701.

# 4 Coexistence of Meniere Disease and Vestibular Migraine

Qing Sun

## 4.1 Summary of Medical Records

Patient, female, 60 years old. Complaint: Recurrent hearing loss in the left ear for 3 years and episodes of vertigo for 1 year. Present history: 3 years ago, the patient suddenly developed hearing loss in the left ear without any obvious cause, and was diagnosed as having sudden deafness at the local hospital. One year ago, the patient had a sudden onset of vertigo with nausea, vomiting, photophobia, and phonophobia, accompanied by increased tinnitus and a feeling of fullness in the left ear, as well as headache and head swelling, and the symptoms lasted for several hours and then her symptoms were relieved by symptomatic treatment. Since then, similar symptoms have recurred, sometimes preceded by a flashing sensation in front of the eyes. In the past 1 month, the patient had frequent episodes of vertigo, averaging two episodes per week, so she was hospitalized for further examination and treatment. Past and family history: The patient had a long-term sleep disorder; no history of hypertension, diabetes mellitus, and hyperlipidemia; no history of motion sickness or migraine; no history of headache or vertigo in family members. Physical examination: No abnormal findings on general and neurological examination. Otologic examination: External auditory canals and tympanic membranes were normal. Pure tone audiometry: Average hearing threshold 56 dBHL in the left ear and 23 dBHL in the right ear. Tympanometry: Both tympanograms were A-shaped curves; stapedial reflex: the reflexes were elicited at all frequencies ipsilateral to the right ear, but not at all frequencies ipsilateral to the left ear. Electrocochleography: Left–SP/AP = 0.45. Auditory brainstem response (ABR) audiometry: Bilateral I-V wave intervals were normal. Vestibular function examination: negative positional test; caloric test showed CP(R) = 10%, indicating normal functions in bilateral horizontal semicircular canals; head shaking nystagmus was seen as rightward horizontal nystagmus with a slow phase nystagmus velocity of 5°/s; cervicogenic vestibular evoked myogenic potential (cVEMP): asymmetry ratio 0.38. Hematological examination: immune function and thyroid function were normal. Brain MRI: no abnormalities were seen. The patient had two episodes of vertigo during his hospitalization. One vertigo episode was accompanied by increased tinnitus, ear fullness, and hearing loss, with fluctuating hearing changes recorded on pure tone audiometry; the other vertigo episode was accompanied by headache and a sensation of flashing light in front of the eyes before the episode. Spontaneous nystagmus was observed in both episodes of vertigo, and the nystagmus was consistent with Alexander's law, but in the

Q. Sun (✉)
Institute of Vertigo, Third Medical Center, PLA General Hospital, Beijing, China

© Scientific and Technical Documentation Press 2023
X. Shan, E. Wang (eds.), *Interpretation of Vertigo Cases*, Experts' Perspectives on Medical Advances, https://doi.org/10.1007/978-981-99-6995-1_4

opposite direction. According to the patient's history and the findings of ancillary tests and examinations, the diagnosis of the co-existence of Meniere disease and vestibular migraine was made and the patient was given the appropriate medication and other conservative treatments for Meniere disease and vestibular migraine, respectively.

## 4.2 Case Study

The patient was a 60-year-old female, with no obvious risk factors for vascular disease indicated in her medical history, and recurrent attacks of hearing loss and vertigo appeared sequentially. Some of the vertigo attacks were accompanied by ear symptoms with definite hearing loss; some of the vertigo attacks were accompanied by headache, head and eye swellings, with visual aura before the vertigo attack. The direction of nystagmus appeared to change during the attack. These two forms of vertigo attacks with individual accompanying symptoms need to be explained by the phenomenon of coexistence of the two diseases (Meniere disease and vestibular migraine). Meniere disease is an idiopathic inner ear disorder in which the main pathological change is endolymphatic hydrops in the membranous labyrinth, and the typical clinical manifestations are recurrent episodes of rotational vertigo, fluctuating hearing loss, tinnitus, and ear fullness. The etiology of Meniere disease remains unclear, and the known causes include the following factors: various infections (bacterial, viral, syphilitic, etc.), injury (including mechanical or acoustic injury), otosclerosis, genetic factors, allergies, tumors, leukemia, and autoimmune diseases. According to the diagnostic criteria for Meniere disease developed by the Barany Society in 2015, Meniere disease may be classified as "definitive Meniere disease" and "probable Meniere disease." The diagnostic criteria for definitive Meniere disease are as follows: (1) $\geq 2$ spontaneous episodes of vertigo, with each vertigo episode lasting between 20 min and 12 h. (2) Audiometrically documented low- to medium-frequency sensorineural hearing loss in one ear, defining the affected ear on at least one occasion before, during, or after one of the episodes of vertigo. (3) Fluctuating auditory symptoms in the affected ear, including hearing loss, tinnitus, or ear fullness. (4) Not better accounted for by another vestibular diagnosis. This patient meets the diagnostic criteria for definitive Meniere disease. According to the diagnostic criteria for vestibular migraine issued by the Barany Society in 2012 and the International Classification of Headache Disorders (ICHD) in 2013, vestibular migraine was also classified as "definitive vestibular migraine" and "probable vestibular migraine." The diagnostic criteria for definitive vestibular migraine were as follows: (1) $\geq 5$ episodes of vestibular symptoms of moderate or severe intensity, lasting between 5 min and 72 h. (2) A present or past history of migraine with or without aura according to ICHD. (3) One or more migraine features with at least 50% of vestibular episodes, such as (a) headache with at least two of the following characteristics: one-sided location, pulsating quality, moderate or severe pain intensity, and aggravation by routine physical activity; (b) photophobia and phonophobia; or (c) visual aura. (4) Not better accounted for by another vestibular or ICHD diagnosis. If a patient meets the above criteria (1), (2) or (3) and (4), they may be diagnosed as probable vestibular migraines. This patient had the symptoms of headache, photophobia, phonophobia, and visual aura, although she had not a definitive history of migraine, thus patient was diagnosed as probable vestibular migraine. Currently, Meniere disease is treated in stages according to its symptoms and degree, with conservative treatment such as medications, and its symptoms such as vertigo can be better controlled in most cases, with a few refractory cases considered for surgical options. Vestibular migraine is mainly treated conservatively with drugs, and its vertigo and headache symptoms can be effectively controlled.

## 4.3 Case Review

Typical symptoms of Meniere disease include a quadruple combination of episodic vertigo, fluctuating sensorineural hearing loss, tinnitus, and a sense of ear fullness, but generally only 50% of patients initially present with both vertigo and hearing loss, 19% with vertigo only, and 26% with deafness only. It is generally accepted that the typical tetralogy should appear 3–5 years after onset. The 1995 edition of the guidelines for the diagnosis and evaluation of therapy in Meniere disease developed by the American Academy of Otolaryngology-Head and Neck Surgery evaluates four frequencies of 0.5, 1, 2, and 3 kHz, with a 20 dBHL increase in mean hearing threshold compared to the contralateral ear for the diagnosis of Meniere disease. While in the diagnostic criteria for Meniere disease developed by the Barany Society, the degree of low-frequency hearing loss was emphasized, in which unilateral lesion is defined as an increase of at least 30 dBHL compared to the contralateral side for two consecutive frequencies below 2 kHz, and bilateral lesions is defined as an increase of 35 dBHL or more for two consecutive frequencies below 2 kHz. The new version of the diagnostic criteria for Meniere disease contains strict limits on the degree of hearing loss, which is very relevant in identifying Meniere disease or vestibular migraine. The pathophysiological relationship between vestibular migraine and Meniere disease is unclear, and it is difficult to distinguish between the two diseases within 1 year of onset, because early Meniere disease may present with only a single vestibular symptom. When the diagnostic criteria for Meniere disease are met, particularly hearing loss confirmed by audiometric testing, the diagnosis of Meniere disease should be made even if migrainous symptoms are present during the attack. Only patients with two different types of attacks, one meeting the criteria for vestibular migraine and one meeting the criteria for Meniere disease, need to be diagnosed with both disorders. Future versions of the International Classification of Headache Disorders (ICHD) may include the coexistence syndrome of vestibular migraine and Meniere disease. The case is characterized by the following two features. (1) Non-coexistence of the tetralogy of Meniere disease. (2) Two forms of vertigo attacks consistent with the coexistence of Meniere disease and vestibular migraine. Clinical recognition and differentiation of such cases is required. Treatment may be pharmacological and conservative for Meniere disease and vestibular migraine, respectively.

## Bibliography

Lopez-Escamez JA, Dlugaiczyk J, Jacobs J, et al. Accompanying symptoms overlap during attacks in Menière's disease and vestibular migraine. Front Neurol. 2014;5:265.

Murofushi T, Tsubota M, Kitao K, et al. Simultaneous presentation of definite vestibular migraine and definite Ménière's disease: overlapping syndrome of two diseases. Front Neurol. 2018;9:749.

Pyykkö I, Manchaiah V, Färkkilä M, et al. Association between Ménière's disease and vestibular migraine. Auris Nasus Larynx. 2019;46(5):724–33.

Shin CH, Kim Y, Yoo MH, et al. Management of Ménière's disease: how does the coexistence of vestibular migraine affect outcomes? Otol Neurotol. 2019;40(5):666–73.

Zhu RT, Van Rompaey V, Ward BK, et al. The interrelations between different causes of dizziness: a conceptual framework for understanding vestibular disorders. Ann Otol Rhinol Laryngol. 2019;128(9):869–78.

# 5 Meniere Disease with Recurrent Sudden Deafness as the Main Manifestation

Haijin Yi

## 5.1 Summary of Medical Records

Patient, male, 65 years old. Complaint: Recurrent hearing loss in the right ear for 8 months. Present history: The patient first visited our hospital 8 months ago due to sudden hearing loss in the right ear after swimming, with symptoms of ear fullness and tinnitus, his tinnitus was buzzing, persistent, obvious in a noisy environment and slightly reduced in a quiet environment, and no complaints of vertigo attacks. On examination at that time: bilateral external auditory canals and tympanic membranes were normal. Patient was admitted to the hospital with a diagnosis of "sudden deafness (right)," and he was treated with methylprednisolone and Ginkgo biloba extract, and the symptoms of tinnitus and fullness in the right ear were basically relieved, and the hearing in the right ear improved. Two months later, following drinking of alcohol, the patient again experienced a significant decrease in hearing in the right ear, with intermittent high-pitched tinnitus and ear fullness, but no vertigo attack, and again consulted our outpatient clinic. The patient was admitted to the hospital with "sudden deafness." Since the patient came to the hospital about 1 month after the onset of the disease, it was considered that prior treatment might not be effective, so he was treated with right tympanotomy tube placement plus intratympanic corticosteroids (dexamethasone 5 mg per injection, 1 injection every 3 days, 4 times in total). After the treatments, the patient's symptoms of right tinnitus and ear fullness were relieved, and the pure tone audiometry showed improvement of hearing: 47.5 dBHL in the right ear, and the patient was discharged. During the following 5 months, the patient had recurrent hearing loss in the right ear, with episodes of right tinnitus, mostly accompanied by a feeling of right ear fullness, and he was seen several times at the outpatient clinic. During the last visit, the patient was asked about his medical history, and he reported that each hearing loss episode was accompanied by vertigo, a sensation of rotating vision, mild nausea, but no vomiting, and a feeling of unsteadiness and walking on cotton, which lasted for several hours and resolved spontaneously. He was admitted to the hospital with "Meniere's disease (right)." Electrocochleography was performed, SP/AP ratio = 0.84. Patient received right endolymphatic sac decompression and right posterior tympanic chamber opening and dexamethasone injection under general anesthesia. One week after surgery, the mean pure tone hearing threshold of the patient's right ear was 43.8 dBHL. Fourteen months after surgery, the patient had no further vertigo attacks and also no further aggravation of hearing loss in the right ear.

H. Yi (✉)
Department of Otolaryngology, Head and Neck Surgery, Beijing Tsinghua Changgung Hospital, Tsinghua University, Beijing, China

© Scientific and Technical Documentation Press 2023
X. Shan, E. Wang (eds.), *Interpretation of Vertigo Cases*, Experts' Perspectives on Medical Advances, https://doi.org/10.1007/978-981-99-6995-1_5

## 5.2 Case Study

Meniere disease is a common otogenic vertigo disorder, and the typical characteristic presenting symptoms at its onset include episodic vertigo, fluctuating hearing loss, tinnitus, and/or a feeling of ear fullness. According to the Chinese Medical Association's 2017 Guidelines for the Diagnosis and Treatment of Meniere's Disease, the diagnostic criteria for Meniere disease are as follows. (1) $\geq$2 episodes of vertigo, each lasting between 20 min and 12 h. (2) At least one audiological examination during the course of the disease confirming low- to medium-frequency sensorineural hearing loss in the affected ear. (3) Fluctuating hearing loss, tinnitus, and/or ear fullness in the affected ear. (4) Exclusion of other diseases causing vertigo. The diagnostic criteria for probable Ménière disease are as follows. (1) $\geq$2 episodes of vertigo, each lasting 20 min to 24 h. (2) Fluctuating hearing loss, tinnitus and/or a feeling of ear fullness in the affected ear. (3) Exclusion of other diseases causing vertigo. In the early stages of Ménière disease, the difference in lesion sites can lead to different clinical presentation of symptoms of Ménière disease, i.e., only cochlear symptoms or vestibular symptoms are present. The concept of "cochlear Ménière's disease" and "vestibular Ménière's disease" was introduced in the 1972 Ménière disease guidelines of the American Academy of Otolaryngology, Head and Neck Surgery. Cochlear Ménière disease is a condition in which the first manifestation of cochlear symptoms is a recurrent sensorineural hearing loss, predominantly at low-to-moderate frequencies, which may be accompanied by a feeling of fullness and tinnitus in the affected ear, with the onset of vertigo months to years later. In recent years, as the understanding of Ménière disease has advanced, "cochlear Ménière's disease" and "vestibular Ménière's disease" are considered to be a reflex of different involving sites of Ménière disease and different stages of disease development, so this concept is rarely used. However, in clinical practice, if we encounter recurrent episodes of fluctuating sensorineural hearing loss, especially in the low and medium frequencies, we need to take carefully a history of vertigo attacks, and if necessary, the examinations of caloric test, vestibular myogenic evoked potentials, electrocochleography, etc. may be taken to assist the diagnosis of this disease.

Treatments of Meniere disease includes treatments during episodes and intermittent treatments. The aims of treatments during the attack phase are to control vertigo attacks, to preserve hearing, and to reduce symptoms. Commonly used medications include vestibular suppressants and glucocorticoids. The aims of intermittent treatments are to reduce, control, or prevent vertigo attacks while preserving the existing inner ear functions, especially hearing function, to the greatest extent possible. Intermittent treatments include both pharmacological and surgical treatments. Treatment medications of Meniere disease generally include betahistine, diuretics, oral glucocorticoids, and intratympanic glucocorticoids or gentamicin. In recent years, intratympanic glucocorticoids have received increasing attention. A randomized, double-blind, controlled clinical study with a 2-year follow-up showed that intratympanic methylprednisolone significantly reduced the number of vertigo episodes, having similar effects to intratympanic gentamicin and significantly less damaging to inner ear function than intratympanic gentamicin. Surgical treatment of Ménière disease generally includes endolymphatic sac surgery, semicircularcanal occlusion, vestibular neurotomy, labyrinthectomy, etc. For patients with stage III Ménière disease, endolymphatic sac surgery is preferred. Traditional endolymphatic sac surgery includes endolymphatic sac decompression and endolymphatic sac drainage. It was reported in the literature that the control rate for vertigo after endolymphatic sac surgery was around 70%, but its long-term efficacy was controversial. In order to improve the surgical efficacy, the combination of endolymphatic sac surgery and intratympanic glucocorticoids has been used in the treatment of Meniere disease in the last decade, including intratympanic glucocorticoids during endolymphatic sac surgery, showing better efficacy than endolymphatic sac surgery only.

## 5.3 Case Review

The clinical manifestations of Ménière disease are varied, and many patients in the early stages do not present with the typical "tetralogy" of episodic vertigo, fluctuating hearing loss, tinnitus, and/or a feeling of ear fullness. Therefore, in clinical practice, patients with recurrent episodes of vertigo lasting between 20 min and 12 h, or fluctuating hearing loss, especially in the low- and medium-frequencies, should be alerted to the possibility of Ménière disease. The diagnosis of Ménière disease is based primarily on history, and therefore detailed history taking is important in patients with suspected Ménière disease. The patient in this case presented with recurrent episodes of hearing loss and was hospitalized several times, but due to the vertigo symptoms in this patient being mild and the history could not be taken carefully by the resident, a timely and correct diagnosis was not obtained. A systemic treatment is required for Meniere disease, of which treatment in remission is key. Control of vertigo attacks and preservation of inner ear function are the two main goals of treatments. Intratympanic glucocorticoids are an option for patients with mild hearing loss in stages I and II, and surgery is an option for patients with frequent vertigo attacks and hearing loss in stages II–IV. This patient had mild vertigo episodes, but his hearing loss reached stage III and also the patient was willing to receive surgical treatment. Endolymphatic sac decompression was performed with opening the posterior tympanic chamber and covering the dexamethasone-soaked gelatin sponge around the round window and on the surface of the endolymphatic sac. Clinical observations showed that the treatments in this patient showed good efficacy for vertigo control and hearing preservation.

## Bibliography

Editorial Board of Chinese Journal of Otolaryngology Head and Neck Surgery, Society of Otolaryngology Head and Neck Surgery, Chinese Medical Association. Guidelines for the diagnosis and treatment of Meniere's disease (2017). Chin J Otolaryngol Head Neck Surg. 2017;52(3):167–72.

Lopez-Escamez JA, Carey J, Chung WH, et al. Diagnostic criteria for Menière's disease. J Vestib Res. 2015;25(1):1–7.

Patel M, Agarwal K, Arshad Q, et al. Intratympanic methylprednisolone versus gentamicin in patients with unilateral Ménière's disease: a randomized, double-blind, comparative effectiveness trial. Lancet. 2016;388(10061):2753–62.

Wick CC, Manzoor NF, McKenna C, et al. Long-term outcomes of endolymphatic sac shunting with local steroids for Meniere's disease. Am J Otolaryngol. 2017;38(3):285–90.

# 6 Meniere Disease with Tumarkin's Crisis

Haijin Yi

## 6.1 Summary of Medical Records

Patient, female, 66 years old. Complaint: Recurrent vertigo attacks for more than 10 years, aggravated for 1 month. Present history: The patient had episodes of vertigo with no obvious cause more than 10 years ago, with rotating vision and nausea, without any obvious hearing loss or tinnitus or ear fullness at that time. The vertigo symptoms were relieved by resting for about 2 h, so no attention was paid and no further treatment was given. Since then, the patient's vertigo symptoms have recurred, once or twice a year. About 3–4 years ago, the symptoms of tinnitus and fullness occurred in the left ear and 2 years ago, these aural symptoms became persistent. And 1 month ago, the patient had another vertigo attack with tipping, which lasted for a few seconds and then relieved, and had three vertigo attacks in the past 1 month, with no significant change in tinnitus, ear fullness, and hearing loss symptoms. The patient had been hospitalized in a local hospital with no significant improvement in symptoms, so she came to our hospital on July 25, 2018. Past history: no history of trauma, and no history of autoimmune disease. No family history of Meniere disease or migraine. Physical examination: general physical condition was good, with no abnormal neurological signs. Otologic examination: Bilateral external auditory canals and tympanic membranes were normal. Pure tone audiometry: both ears showed sensorineural hearing loss, with predominantly in low to medium frequency and more severe in the left ear (Fig. 6.1). Tympanometry: both ears showed type A tympanogram. Electrocochleography: left ear−SP/AP = 0.32. Vestibular function examination: saccade test was normal; smooth pursuit test was type II curve; the optokinetic test showed normal and symmetrical optokinetic nystagmus bilaterally. Gaze test was not abnormal. Spontaneous nystagmus and positional tests were negative; the Dix-Hallpike test and supine roll test were negative; caloric test: the maximum slow phase velocity of nystagmus was 1–4°/s for cool or warm water stimulation in both ears, respectively, indicating bilateral reduced horizontal semicircular canal functions. Clinical diagnosis: Based on the patient's symptoms and ancillary examination findings, a diagnosis of Meniere disease (left) with Tumarkin's crisis was made. Treatment: the patient was treated with surgery to improve her vertigo symptoms in view of the poor results of conservative treatment. Patient underwent left tympanotomy tube placement under local anesthesia on July 30, 2018, with intraoperative dexamethasone injection of 5 mg/mL via the tympanic ventricular tube. Thereafter the patient was generally well, with occasional vertigo symptoms. On the third and

H. Yi (✉)
Department of Otolaryngology, Head and Neck Surgery, Beijing Tsinghua Changgung Hospital, Tsinghua University, Beijing, China

© Scientific and Technical Documentation Press 2023
X. Shan, E. Wang (eds.), *Interpretation of Vertigo Cases*, Experts' Perspectives on Medical Advances, https://doi.org/10.1007/978-981-99-6995-1_6

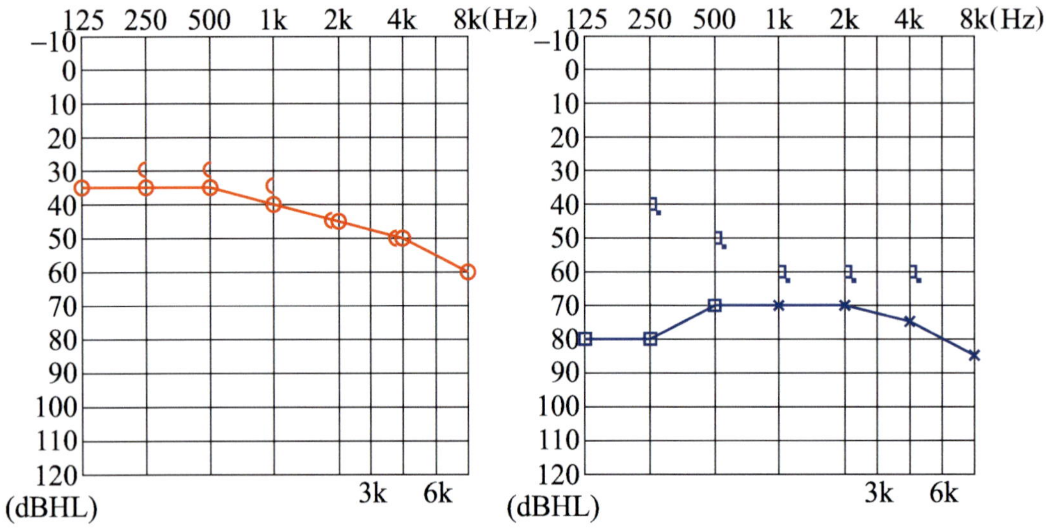


**Fig. 6.1** Pure tone audiometry: sensorineural hearing loss in both ears, severer in the left ear

seventh postoperative days, respectively, 40 mg/mL of methylprednisolone was injected in the left tympanic chamber under endoscopy, and there was no bleeding or signs of infection in the ear. The patient was discharged the next day. The patient has not had any further attacks of vertigo or Tumarkin's crisis during the postoperative 4-month follow-up by telephone.

## 6.2 Case Study

Patient was an elderly female with Meniere disease, whose early symptoms were atypical, showing only recurrent episodes of vertigo without significant hearing loss and symptoms of tinnitus and ear fullness, and the cochlear symptoms of tinnitus, ear fullness, and hearing loss appeared after several years of vertigo attacks. This may be the main reason why this patient did not receive a timely and definitive diagnosis at an early stage and the possible reason why she was not given attention and further treatment. Based on the patient's medical history, clinical symptoms, examination findings, and current diagnostic criteria for Meniere disease, the patient was diagnosed with Meniere disease (left) with Tumarkin's crisis. The patient also presented with mild to moderate sensorineural deafness in the right ear, the cause of which was unknown, and the diagnosis of bilateral Meniere disease could not be ruled out at this time. The patient was admitted to the hospital for receiving tympanotomy tube placement as well as tympanic dexamethasone injection because of the poor results of conservative treatment, and the patient's vertigo symptoms basically were resolved after treatments. Follow-up of the patient was intensified to observe the long-term treatment effect and to further clarify the presence of bilateral Meniere disease.

## 6.3 Case Review

Meniere disease is a common peripheral vertiginous disorder. It is an inner ear disease of unknown cause, with endolymphatic hydrops in the membranous labyrinth as the main pathological feature and episodic vertigo, fluctuating hearing loss, tinnitus, and/or ear fullness as typical clinical manifestations. The etiology and pathogenesis of Meniere disease are still not well understood. It is generally believed that the pathogenesis of Meniere disease is the result of the involvement of multiple factors, including genetic and environmental factors, and its triggers include tiredness, stress and mood change, sleep disorders, adverse life events, and weather or seasonal condition. Tumarkin's crisis (vestibular drop attack), also known as otolithic crisis, is a vertigo attack accompanied by a sudden fall that lasts for a few seconds and occurs only in the standing position, with no signs before the fall and most often without loss of consciousness. Tumarkin's crisis is a rare phenomenon, usually associated with advanced Meniere disease.

In 2015, the Barany Society published new diagnostic criteria for Meniere disease, which have been widely adopted, and the Chinese Society of Otolaryngology, Head and Neck Surgery and the European Academy of Otology and Neurotology have newly published corresponding guidelines for the management of Meniere disease. There is no specific treatment or prevention method for Meniere disease, and it is usually treated conservatively with medication and surgery. Drug therapy is based on systemic medication, which has a low control rate of vertigo and no therapeutic effect on hearing damage. In recent years, the treatment of Meniere disease by intratympanic injection of steroid hormones has received increasing attention and has become an important route of administration for the treatment of Meniere disease. The effect is better than that of systemic administration because only a small amount of the drug diffuses into the bloodstream, which can avoid or reduce the adverse effects of systemic administration and is suitable for patients who have contraindications to systemic hormone application. Since Meniere disease may be associated with allergic or autoimmune disorders, glucocorticoids are of therapeutic value in patients with Meniere disease. These hormones act through the glucocorticoid receptors present in the inner ear, and their mechanisms of action are not fully understood, including neuroprotection, inhibiting apoptosis, increasing cochlear blood flow, and reducing endolymphatic hydrops. A prospective placebo-controlled randomized clinical trial showed that, after treatment with intratympanic dexamethasone, 82% patients obtained complete control of vertigo, 48% with improvement in subjective tinnitus, 35% with improvement in hearing, and 48% with improvement in ear fullness, all of which were significantly better than those inpatients of control group. It was found in another study that repeat intratympanic dexamethasone in patients for whom initial intratympanic dexamethasone ineffective offered a Class A control rate of 15.7%. Intratympanic dexamethasone was also effective in controlling episodes of vertigo in delayed endolymphatic hydrops and reduced effectively the episodes of falls in advanced stages of Meniere disease. Thus, in patients with Meniere disease who have failed to respond to conservative drug therapy, intratympanic glucocorticoids can achieve high vertigo control rates with few adverse effects, and it can be used as an alternative therapy when oral drug therapy is ineffective or when systemic medication is not available because of contraindications. This treatment preserves both cochlear function and vestibular function of patients.

The patient's symptoms were atypical in the early stage and thus she was not clearly diagnosed in time, and also was not given specific attention and further treatment. Recently, the vertigo attacks became frequent and severe, even with Tumarkin's crisis, and also the hearing loss was worsening in the patient. The patient was treated with tympanotomy tube placement plus intraoperative and postoperative intratympanic glucocorticoids, showing good treatment efficacy. The long-term effect of the treatment remains to be evaluated.

## Bibliography


Editorial Board of Chinese Journal of Otolaryngology, Head and Neck Surgery, Society of Otolaryngology Head and Neck Surgery, Chinese Medical Association. Guidelines for the diagnosis and treatment of Meniere disease (2017). Chin J Otolaryngol Head Neck Surg. 2017;52(3):167–72.

Frejo L, Martin-Sanz E, Teggi R, et al. Extended phenotype and clinical subgroups in unilateral Meniere disease: a cross-sectional study with cluster analysis. Clin Otolaryngol. 2017;42(6):1172–80.

Lopez-Escamez JA, Carey J, Chung WH, et al. Diagnostic criteria for Menière's disease. J Vestib Res. 2015;25(1):1–7.

Magnan J, Ozgirgin ON, Trabalzini F, et al. European position statement on diagnosis, and treatment of Meniere's disease. J Int Adv Otol. 2018;14(2):317–21.

Patel M, Agarwal K, Arshad Q, et al. Intratympanic methylprednisolone versus gentamicin in patients with unilateral Ménière's disease: a randomised, double-blind, comparative effectiveness trial. Lancet. 2016;388(10061):2753–62.

# 7 Immune-Responsive Meniere Disease

Li Zhang

## 7.1 Summary of Medical Records

Patient, female, 68 years old, Mongolian ethnicity. Complaint: Seasonal sneezing and runny nose with tinnitus, hearing loss, and vertigo attacks for more than 5 years. Present history: The patient started to have seasonal allergic rhinitis symptoms such as sneezing and runny nose 5 years ago, and the symptoms worsened in May every year when the flowers bloom, and had tinnitus in the left ear at the same time. The more severe the tinnitus symptoms, the more severe the dizziness symptoms. These symptoms usually resolved by the end of October, but in the following year, around mid-May, similar symptoms started to appear again, and have continued for more than 5 years now. Pure tone audiometry: hearing loss in both ears with a tendency to deteriorate year by year, more severe hearing loss in the left ear, and predominant in low frequency. Vestibular function tests: spontaneous nystagmus, gaze nystagmus, and positional nystagmus were all negative, saccade test and smooth pursuit test were normal, caloric test showed stronger nystagmus response in the left ear than that in the right ear, with directional preponderance = 55%. Allergen testing: allergy to house dust, but no clear allergy to typical Inner Mongolian allergens such as Artemisia and Humulus was found. The diagnosis was allergic rhinitis and immunoreactive Meniere disease. Treatment: (1) Oral montelukast sodium (10 mg, once daily). (2) Physiologic seawater nasal spray and mometasone furoate nasal spray. (3) Oral betahistine mesylate tablets (12 mg, 3 times a day). (4) Oral spironolactone and hydrochlorothiazide (1 tablet each, once daily in the morning). (5) Intravenous Kinardol (105 mg, once daily). After 1 week of treatment, the patient's dizziness symptom resolved and her hearing improved.

## 7.2 Case Study

The patient, an elderly female of Mongolian ethnicity, complained of seasonal sneezing, runny nose, and other symptoms of allergic rhinitis with tinnitus, hearing loss, and vertigo episodes for the past 5 years, and her vertigo and aural symptoms were reduced when her symptoms of allergic rhinitis were controlled. These symptoms usually resolved by the end of October, but the following year, around mid-May, similar symptoms started again and have persisted for more than 5 years now. Pure tone audiometry showed that the patient's hearing decreased in both ears and tended to decrease year by year, and the hearing loss in the left ear was more severe, with low-frequency hearing loss predominating, consistent with the hearing manifestations of Meniere's

L. Zhang (✉)
Department of Otolaryngology, Head and Neck Surgery, Affiliated Hospital of Inner Mongolia Medical University, Hohhot, China

© Scientific and Technical Documentation Press 2023

X. Shan, E. Wang (eds.), *Interpretation of Vertigo Cases*, Experts' Perspectives on Medical Advances, https://doi.org/10.1007/978-981-99-6995-1_7

disease. The vestibular function test showed that spontaneous nystagmus, gaze nystagmus, and positional nystagmus were all negative, and the saccade test and smooth pursuit test were also normal. Caloric test showed a stronger nystagmus response in the left ear than in the right, and directinal preponderance was 55%. Allergen testing showed the allergy to house dust, but clear allergies to typical Inner Mongolian allergens such as Artemisia and Humulus were not found. Based on the patient's history and clinical presentation, she was considered to have both seasonal allergic rhinitis and Meniere disease, and the latter should be immunoreactive Meniere disease. Therefore, in addition to treating the patient accordingly for Meniere disease, the patient should be treated aggressively for allergic rhinitis to suppress the allergic reaction. After systematic treatment, the patient's allergic rhinitis was controlled, dizziness was gradually relieved, and hearing improved.

## 7.3 Case Review

Meniere disease is a common condition in otolaryngology and one of the most common causes of peripheral vertigo. The incidence of Meniere disease varies widely among countries, regions, and ethnic groups. A multicenter study in Japan in 1995 reported a prevalence of 16/100,000, and in 2007, the United States reported a prevalence of 190/100,000. Meniere disease is characterized by recurrent episodes of vertigo, fluctuating hearing loss, tinnitus, and a sense of ear fullness as the main clinical manifestations. Fluctuating low-frequency sensorineural hearing loss is one of the features of early cochlear lesions in Meniere disease. As the disease progresses, the low-frequency hearing loss gradually worsens and progresses to the middle and high frequency bands, and in the late stage of Meniere disease, patients may manifest as moderate to severe non-fluctuating hearing loss in the full frequency band. At present, the diagnosis of Meniere disease is mainly based on the patient's medical history and clinical symptoms. The clinical staging of Meniere disease and clinical treatment are based on the degrees of the hearing loss.

The etiology and pathogenesis of Meniere disease are still not well understood. Various theories have been proposed regarding its etiology and pathogenesis, including the theory of mechanical obstruction of the endolymphatic duct and impaired endolymphatic absorption, the theory of immune response, and the theory of inner ear ischemia. It is generally believed that the development of Meniere disease may be related to an imbalance between endolymphatic production and absorption, resulting in endolymphatic hydrops in the membranous labyrinth. The endolymphatic sac is a key site for causing immune responses in the inner ear, and disturbances in its immune activity may contribute to the development of Meniere disease and vertigo attacks. Meniere disease is closely related to allergic reactions. In 1923, Duke first reported two cases of Meniere disease in patients with food allergy and postulated that the mechanisms of pathogenesis of Meniere disease by allergic reactions and immune abnormalities are as follows: (1) Contact immune reaction, i.e., when direct contact or ingestion of allergens caused a direct reaction between the antigens and antibodies, resulting in allergic damage to the inner ear; (2) Systemic immune response, i.e., patients had a systemic allergic disease, where Meniere disease was a local manifestation of the disease. Subsequently, a controlled trial revealed that the positive rate of allergen testing in patients with Meniere disease was significantly higher than the average positive rate of allergen testing in general population in the same region, and there was a strong correlation between seasonal allergic reactions and circulating immune complexes. This case was a Mongolian patient with Meniere disease, whose episodes of Meniere disease were accompanied by the onset of seasonal allergic rhinitis, which was thought to be caused by an immune disorder involving the endolymphatic sacs, namely the inner ear immune organ, and the patient should be treated with appropriate therapy for the concomitant immune disorder in order to achieve effective control of Meniere disease and vertigo attacks.

## Bibliography

Editorial Board of Chinese Journal of Otolaryngology Head and Neck Surgery, Society of Otolaryngology Head and Neck Surgery, Chinese Medical Association. Guidelines for the diagnosis and treatment of Meniere's disease (2017). Chin J Otolaryngol Head Neck Surg. 2017;52(3):167–72.

Platt M, Dilwali S, Elackattu A, et al. Mining immune epitopes in the inner ear. Otolaryngol Head Neck Surg. 2014;150(3):460–3.

# 8 Vestibular Neuritis (Acute Unilateral Vestibulopathy)

Hui Leng

## 8.1 Summary of Medical Records

Patient, male, 73 years old. Chief complaint: acute vertigo attack for 1 day. Present history: The patient began to have significant vertigo symptoms 1 day ago, with a sensation of rotation of vision, aggravated by change of body position, with nausea and vomiting symptoms, he was conscious, without symptoms of hearing loss, tinnitus and ear fullness, and was seen on September 25, 2018 because the vertigo symptoms persisted without relief. Past history: no previous history of vertigo attacks, no recent history of upper respiratory tract infection or fever. Physical examination: temperature 36.2 °C, cooperative for examination, no enlargement of superficial lymph nodes, no abnormalities in heart, lung, abdomen, and limb examinations. Neurological system: normal muscle strength and tone of the extremities, normal tendon reflexes, negative bilateral Babinski's signs, and negative finger-nose test, alternating test and heel-knee-shin test. Otological examination: both external ear canals and ear drums were normal. Head impulse test: positive rightward head impulse test (HIT). Pure tone audiometry: high frequency hearing loss in both ears (Fig. 8.1). Nystagmography: positive spontaneous nystagmus with leftward horizontal nystagmus and a maximum slow phase velocity of 8.0°/s. The optokinetic test was normal. Video HIT (vHIT): suggesting impaired vestibular oculomotor reflex (VOR) pathways in the right horizontal semicircular canal and right anterior semicircular canal (Fig. 8.2). The cervical vestibular-evoked myogenic potential (cVEMP) test was normal. Static eye rotation test: 20° in the right eye and 3° in the left eye (Fig. 8.3). Head tilt test: positive (tilt to the right). Subjective visual vertical line (SVV): −8.9°. Subjective visual horizontal line (SVH): −11.1°. No abnormalities on cranial MRI, DWI, and MRA. Diagnosis: vestibular neuritis (right superior vestibular neuritis), also called as acute unilateral vestibulopathy. Treatments: (1) Sedation, antiemetic, and antivertigo symptomatic treatments, e.g., isoprostanes 25 mg, intramuscularly, once daily. (2) Glucocorticoids, such as prednisone 60 mg/day, morning dose, tapered after 4 days. (3) Drugs for improving blood supply and nutrition of nerve, such as Ginkgo biloba extract and neurotrophic factor. (4) After 3 days, the patient's nystagmus was reduced, and he was encouraged to get up and to perform vestibular rehabilitation exercises to obtain vestibular compensation as soon as possible. Vestibular rehabilitation exercises: walking exercises, 10 min each time, 3 times a day; gaze stabilization exercises: horizontal, vertical, and diagonal head movement exercises, 20–30 times each, once a day. (5) Acupuncture: 30 min each time, including

H. Leng (✉)
Department of Otolaryngology, Affiliated Hospital of Liaoning Traditional Chinese Medicine University, Shenyang, China

© Scientific and Technical Documentation Press 2023

X. Shan, E. Wang (eds.), *Interpretation of Vertigo Cases*, Experts' Perspectives on Medical Advances, https://doi.org/10.1007/978-981-99-6995-1_8

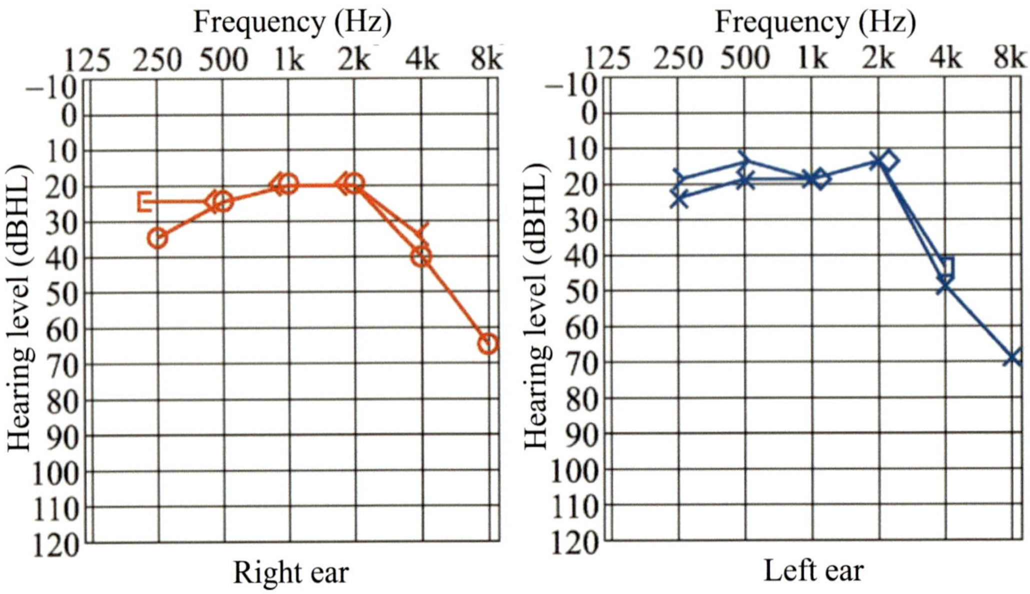


**Fig. 8.1** Pure tone audiometry. High frequency hearing loss in both ears

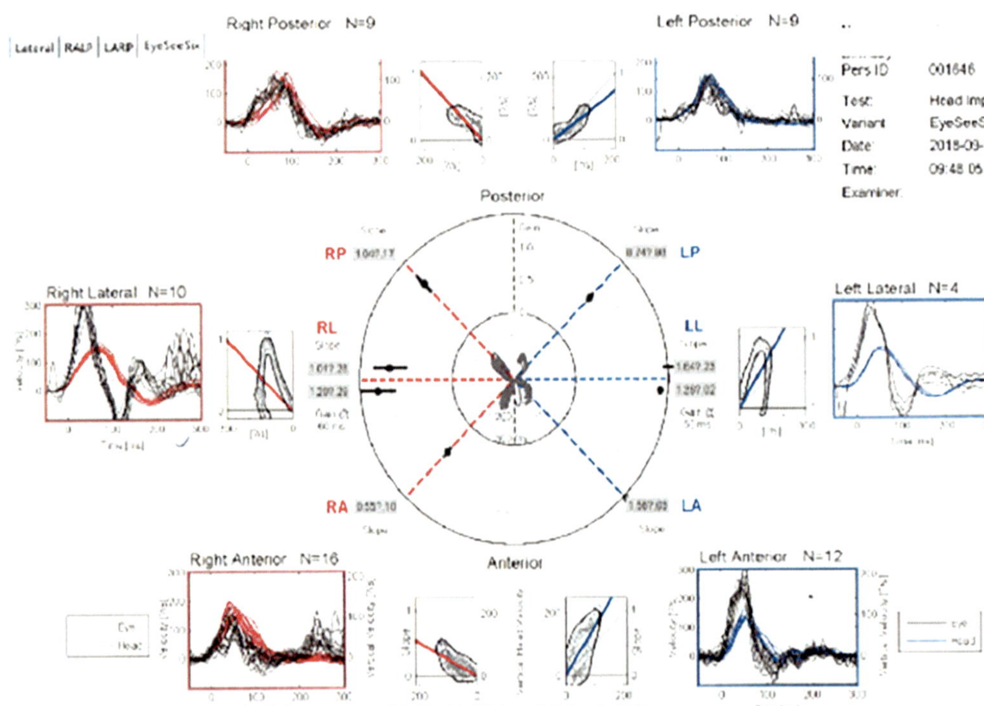


**Fig. 8.2** Video head impulse test (vHIT). It was indicated that vestibular oculomotor reflex (VOR) pathways of the right horizontal and anterior semicircular canals were impaired

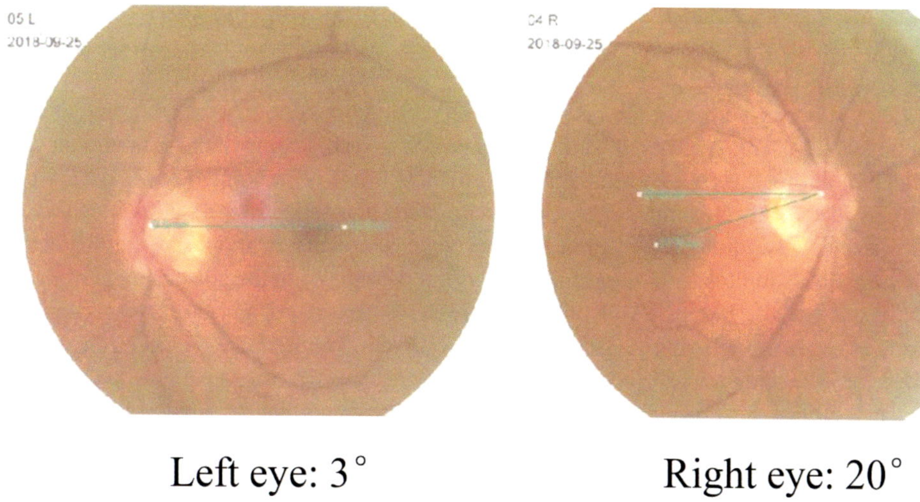


**Fig. 8.3** Static eye rotation test

bilateral Taiyang, Yintang and Baihui acupuncture points as well as dizzy-hearing area. On the fourth day of treatment, the patient's vertigo symptoms were reduced, no more nausea or vomiting occurred, and the spontaneous nystagmus was gradually reduced. On the seventh day of treatment, the patient felt his vertigo symptoms were significantly reduced, with no visual rotation, but still a floating sensation, and the spontaneous nystagmus disappeared, and the review of vestibular function showed that the spontaneous nystagmus became negative. After 2 weeks of treatment, the patient's vertigo symptoms basically disappeared and he was discharged with clinical symptoms relieved.

## 8.2 Case Study

The patient is an elderly male who presented with an acute vertigo attack for 1 day without cochlear symptoms such as hearing loss, tinnitus, and a feeling of ear fullness. Pure tone audiometry: high frequency hearing loss in both ears. Nystagmography: positive spontaneous nystagmus showing leftward horizontal nystagmus with a maximum slow phase velocity of 8.0°/s. HIT: positive rightward HIT. vHIT suggested the damages to the right horizontal semicircular canal and right anterior semicircular canal VOR pathways. Static eye rotation test: 20° in the right eye, 3° in the left eye. Positive head tilt test (tilt to the right). SVV: −8.9°. SVH: −11.1°. The patient had no other positive neurological signs, and no abnormalities were seen on brain MRI, DWI, and MRA. According to the patient's history, clinical presentation, and relevant findings, he was diagnosed with vestibular neuritis (right superior vestibular neuritis). The diagnosis of the disease was based on: (1) Acute or subacute onset, presenting with persistent rotational vertigo and nausea and vomiting, with horizontal spontaneous nystagmus. (2) Absence of symptoms of tinnitus and hearing loss. (3) Absence of other neurological signs or symptoms suggestive of central nervous system diseases. (4) Caloric test showing hyporesponsiveness or unresponsiveness on one side. The combination of VEMP and vHIT findings allows for the classification of vestibular neuritis into three subtypes: superior vestibular neuritis, inferior vestibular neuritis, and total vestibular neuritis. Superior vestibular neuritis: vHIT shows decreased gain in the affected superior and horizontal semicircular canals, with abnormal oVEMP and normal cVEMP on the affected side. Inferior vestibular neuritis: vHIT presents with decreased gain in the affected posterior semicircular canal, abnormal cVEMP on the affected side, and normal oVEMP. Total vestibular neuritis: vHIT presents with decreased gain in the affected three semicircular canals and abnormal oVEMP and cVEMP on the affected side. In the process of diagnosis for vestibular neuritis, it should be differentiated from Meniere disease. The diagnostic criteria for Meniere disease are as follows: (1) ≥2 episodes of vertigo, each lasting between 20 min and 12 h. (2) At least one audiometric examination during the course of the disease confirming low- and medium-frequency sensorineural hearing loss in the affected ear. (3) Fluctuating hearing loss, tinnitus, and/or ear fullness in the affected ear. (4) Exclusion of other diseases causing vertigo, including vestibular neuritis. Based on the diagnostic criteria for Meniere disease described above, vestibular neuritis is not difficult to differentiate from Meniere disease. The disease also needs to be differentiated from central vertigo. Studies of isolated cerebellar infarction cases have shown that 10% of patients have a clinical presentation similar to vestibular neuritis. Brain MRI is required when infarction is clinically suspected. This case could be largely excluded from having central vertigo by brain MRI.

For the treatments of vestibular neuritis, if acute vertigo episodes are severe at the beginning of the disease, intramuscular isoprostanes are given as antiemetic and antivertigo symptomatic treatment. This class of drugs has negative effect on the formation of vestibular center compensations, so they are no longer used after acute symptoms are reduced. Hormones are currently the drugs of choice in the clinical treatment of vestibular neuritis. They play a therapeutic role by promoting the recovery of peripheral vestibular function and accelerating central vestibular compensation, which can directly activate the neurons of the medial vestibular nucleus and accelerate vestibular compensation. The therapeutic effect of hormones is also derived from their anti-inflammatory effect, i.e., they may improve peripheral vestibular function by reducing tissue swelling in the vestibular nerve and inner ear vestibule. Vestibular rehabilitation therapy (VRT) is a physical approach to the treatment of central and peripheral balance disorders that was first proposed by Cooksey and Cawthorne in the 1940s, but has not received much attention until recently. It can be used in patients with unilateral or bilateral vestibular impairment to reduce dizziness, improve balance function, reduce the risk of falls, improve vestibular oculomotor reflexes, enhance gait stability, and reduce anxiety symptoms due to vertigo. Some studies suggest that VRT is comparable to treatment with hormones. It has been pointed out that the treatment of vestibular neuritis requires a change in the emphasis on medication and the neglect of physical therapy. With the advancement of medical research on vertigo, it is gradually recognized that vestibular compensation is a central process, and the treatment of such patients is changing from purely symptomatic treatment to promoting central compensation. Pharmacological treatment can reduce the symptoms and promote vestibular compensation after vestibular damage. Ginkgo preparations may directly counteract necrosis and neuronal apoptosis and enhance neuronal plasticity such as vestibular compensation by following mechanisms: (1) Changes of histological structures in the vestibular nucleus system, associated with increased synaptic structures and enhanced function in the vestibular nucleus region. (2) Association with the vestibular nucleus system excitatory neurotransmitter glutamate and its receptor N-methyl-D-aspartate receptor (NMDA) subunit $R_1$, with the recovery of both in the process of compensation. (3) Astrocytes of the vestibular nucleus system affect vestibular compensation or protect vestibular nucleus neurons in some ways. (4) Ginkgo preparations have a protective effect on vestibular ganglia, and delayed metaplasia may also affect vestibular compensation. Neurotrophic metabolic agents are now also commonly used in the treatment of vestibular neuritis, such as vitamin $B_1$, vitamin $B_{12}$, sodium cytarabine, sodium tetrahexose monosialate ganglioside injection, nerve growth factors, and olanzapine to improve the metabolic processes of damaged nerves.

## 8.3 Case Review

Vestibular neuritis, also known as acute unilateral vestibulopathy, is characterized by acute unilateral vestibular hypofunction or dysfunction. In 1909, Ruttin first reported a disease with sudden attacks of vertigo without cochlear or other neurological symptoms, and in 1924, Nylen called the disease vestibular neuritis. Schuknecht, with histopathological studies, revealed the disease damaged both the vestibular nerve and peripheral receptors. The etiology of the disease is still not well understood and there are several theories. (1) Viral infection. Thirty percent of patients have a history of cold or upper respiratory tract infection before the onset of the disease, or it occurs during an epidemic period of a certain virus, so it is presumed that the disease is caused by viral infection of the vestibular nerve. It is believed that there are two possible mechanisms of virus-induced damage to the vestibular nerve and vestibular ganglia: one is direct infection, and another one is post-infection immune damage. And two models for viral injury have also been proposed: one model is vestibular neuritis caused by pathogenic bacteria originating in the respiratory tract; another model is that the onset of vestibular neuritis in association with activation of dormant herpes simplex virus type I (HSV). (2) Focal infection. This can follow acute or chronic inflammations of the nose, sinuses, tonsils, gastrointestinal tract, biliary tract, or urinary tract, resulting in vestibular nerve infection or edema due to an allergic reaction of the nerve tissue to bacterial endotoxins. (3) Vascular factors. Circulatory disturbances in the small arteries feeding the vestibular nerve may be a cause of the disease. (4) Diabetes mellitus. It is believed that diabetes can cause degenerative atrophy of vestibular neurons, leading to recurrent vertigo attacks. One study showed that 68.4% of diabetic patients with vestibular hypofunction, indicating that diabetic patients may have functional abnormalities of the vestibular nervous system. Pathological examination in some patients with vestibular neuritis after vestibular nerve dissection showed isolated or scattered degeneration and regeneration of the vestibular nerves, with decreased nerve fibers, formation of ganglion cell vacuoles, and increased collagen deposits in the nerves.

In 2001, Aw first described inferior vestibular neuritis. Currently, vestibular neuritis can be divided into subtypes such as total vestibular neuritis, superior vestibular neuritis, and inferior vestibular neuritis. Superior vestibular neuritis is the most common, followed by total vestibular neuritis, and inferior vestibular neuritis is less common, which may be related to the fact that the superior vestibular nerve travels in a longer bony canal to make it more prone to ischemia and edema. In 1993, Ogata reported a case of bilateral vestibular neuritis. An epidemiological study showed that the prevalence of bilateral vestibular neuritis was 5.3%. Because of bilateral vestibular neuropathy, patients may not present with typical vertigo symptoms but often complain of balance disorders, so clinical attention should be paid to screening. This case received a prompt and definitive diagnosis and appropriate systemic treatments. The patient's clinical symptoms were gradually relieved, and his vertigo symptoms basically disappeared after 2 weeks of treatment.

## Bibliography

Arnold SA, Stewart AM, Moor HM, et al. The effectiveness of vestibular rehabilitation interventions in treating unilateral peripheral vestibular disorders: a systematic review. Physiother Res Int. 2017;22(3):e1635. https://doi.org/10.1002/pri.1635.

Deveze A, Bernard-Demanze L, Xavier F, et al. Vestibular compensation and vestibular rehabilitation. Current concepts and new trends. Neurophysiol Clin. 2014;44(1):49–57.

Goudakos JK, Markou KD, Psillas G, et al. Corticosteroids and vestibular exercises in vestibular neuritis: single-blind randomized clinical trial. JAMA Otolaryngol Head Neck Surg. 2014;140(5):434–40.

Hall CD, Herdman SJ, Whitney SL, et al. Vestibular rehabilitation for peripheral vestibular hypofunction: an evidence-based clinical practice guideline: from the American Physical Therapy Association Neurology Section. J Neurol Phys Ther. 2016;40(2):124–55.

Whitney SL, Alghadir AH, Anwer S. Recent evidence about the effectiveness of vestibular rehabilitation. Curr Treat Options Neurol. 2016;18(3):13.

# Bilateral Vestibulopathy

# 9

Lei Zhang and Yuanxing Chen

## 9.1 Summary of Medical Records

Patient, female, 65 years old. Complaint: Hearing loss in both ears, tinnitus, and dizziness for 3 years. Present history: The patient began to experience hearing loss in both ears 3 years ago, which was progressive and accompanied by tinnitus, but was not treated. About a few months later, she started to experience dizziness, which was persistent, with no sensation of rotation of visual objects, relieved by bed rest and aggravated by activity, accompanied by unstable walking, blurred vision when walking, unstable walking in dark environment, without nausea or vomiting, no photophobia or phonophobia, no visual aura such as flashing lights or bright spots in front of the eyes, and no symptoms of blackness, diplopia, dysarthria, and impaired consciousness. The patient had symptoms of unsteadiness in standing, swaying and wanting to fall, and needed support to walk. Past history: having a history of hypertension for 20 years, taking oral nifedipine extended-release tablets, 20 mg each time, once daily, with blood pressure controlled at about 150/95 mmHg; a history of diabetes mellitus for 4 months, taking oral metformin tablets, 0.5 g each time, 3 times daily, with unknown glycemic control; having cerebral infarction 4 years ago, with no significant sequelae; diagnosed as "vertebral artery stenosis" in another hospital and underwent vertebral artery stenting surgery 3 months ago, but her symptoms did not improve after the surgery. Physical examination: showing clear consciousness, fluent speech, tangential answers, bilateral limb muscle strength at grade V, normal pain and temperature sensation, normal knee tendon reflexes on two sides, Romberg's sign (+), bilateral Babinski's sign (−). Otological examination: negative spontaneous nystagmus, no abnormalities in the bilateral external auditory canals, tympanic membrane, and mastoid area. Tuning fork test: bilateral Lintner's tests (RT) (+); Weber's test (WT), centered; Schwabacher's test (ST) (±). Pure tone audiometry: right ear hearing thresholds 30 dBHL/0.5 kHz, 35 dBHL/1 kHz, 40 dBHL/2 kHz, and 60 dBHL/4 kHz, respectively, with a mean hearing threshold of 41.3 dBHL; left ear hearing thresholds 25 dBHL/0.5 kHz, 25 dBHL/1 kHz, 40 dBHL/2 kHz, and 60 dBHL/4 kHz, with a mean hearing threshold of 37.5 dBHL. Tympanometry: normal type A tympanograms in two ears. Acoustic reflexes were elicited at 1 kHz ipsilateral to the right ear and 0.5, 1, and 2 kHz ipsilateral to the left ear. Auditory brainstem-evoked potentials: binaural

L. Zhang
Head and Neck Rehabilitation Center, Beijing Rehabilitation Hospital, Capital Medical University, Beijing, China

Y. Chen (✉)
Institute of Vertigo, Third Medical Center, PLA General Hospital, Beijing, China

© Scientific and Technical Documentation Press 2023

X. Shan, E. Wang (eds.), *Interpretation of Vertigo Cases*, Experts' Perspectives on Medical Advances, https://doi.org/10.1007/978-981-99-6995-1_9

thresholds of 50 dBnHL, good differentiation of each wave, and normal I-V wave intervals. Vestibular function examination: spontaneous nystagmus (−); positional test (−); optokinetic test (−); caloric test: no response to cool and warm water stimulation of the horizontal semicircular canals bilaterally; and rotation test: no significant nystagmus was elicited bilaterally. The clinical diagnosis was bilateral vestibulopathy (BVP). Treatment and results: After treatments with vestibular rehabilitation and drugs to improve microcirculation and nerve nutrition, the patient's balance symptoms improved significantly and she could walk without support.

## 9.2 Case Study

The patient had a slow onset with progressive development of symptoms for up to 3 years, with typical symptoms of unsteadiness in walking and oscillopsia during movement, which were aggravated in the dark environment. The caloric test and rotation test did not induce significant nystagmus, suggesting that the patient had severe bilateral vestibular hypofunction, and pure tone audiometry showed bilateral sensorineural deafness, considering that the patient had vestibular and cochlear neuropathy and dysfunction, and combined with the above history and clinical manifestations, the patient was diagnosed with BVP, and his diagnosis was also in accordance with the diagnostic criteria for BVP published by the Barany Society in 2017. (1) The disease is a chronic vestibular syndrome with the following symptoms: (a) symptoms of unsteadiness when walking or standing, with at least symptom b and/or symptom c; (b) symptoms of motion-induced blurred vision or oscillopsia when walking or during rapid head and body movements; (c) worsening of symptoms of unsteadiness in dark environments and/or on uneven ground. (2) No symptoms when sitting or lying at rest. (3) Bilateral reduced or absent vestibular oculomotor reflex (VOR) function confirmed by video head impulse test (vHIT) or nystagmography: bilateral pathologically reduced VOR gain in vHIT of horizontal canals, <0.6 at two sides; and/or reduced caloric response (sum of maximum slow phase velocity of nystagmus on each side <6°/s); and/or reduced horizontal angular VOR gain <0.1 on sinusoidal stimulation on rotatory chair test (0.1 Hz, $V_{max}$ = 50°/s) and a phase lead ≥15°(time constant ≤6 s). (4) Cannot be better explained by other diseases. A clear history of primary disease in the patient was not indicated with careful history taking. Because of the combination of hypertension, diabetes mellitus, and a history of cerebral infarction in the patient, it was considered that the patient's bilateral vestibular and cochlear lesions were probably due to vascular factors. The patient was given the following treatment. (1) Educating the patient on the possible causes of the disease, types of disease, pathogenesis, causes of symptoms, disease process, and outcome. (2) Giving the patient targeted vestibular rehabilitation exercises to accelerate adaptation to the loss of vestibular function by promoting central compensation and visual and proprioceptive substitution. (3) Promoting the rehabilitation of the patient's vestibular function by giving pharmacological treatments such as improving the microcirculation and nutrition of nerves. With these treatments, the patient's balance disorder symptoms gradually improved.

## 9.3 Case Review

BVP is a chronic vestibular syndrome characterized by postural and gait instability when walking or standing, with insidious onset and slow progression, making it easy to be underdiagnosed or misdiagnosed. BVP can affect children to the elderly, and the age of onset is usually 50–60 years old, and the average age at diagnosis is 62 years old. Most patients with BVP have an unknown cause, and only some patients have a definite or probable cause, with ototoxic drugs, bilateral Meniere disease, and meningitis being the most common causes.

Patients with BVP can suffer from the dysfunctions of VOR and vestibulospinal reflex due to the damage or function loss of bilateral vestibular afferent nerves. As a result of VOR deficiency, images on the retina cannot be presented stably during rapid head movements and swaying occurs, with symptoms such as head movement-induced oscillopsia, dynamic vision loss, and blurred vision. Due to the absence of vestibulospinal reflexes, patients may experience symptoms of postural and gait instability during walking and standing due to impaired postural balance control. Since the visual and proprioceptive systems are also involved in maintaining body balance, postural balance dysfunction can be exacerbated when BVP patient's postural control is not adequately compensated by proprioceptive information afferents (e.g., on soft or uneven ground) or visual information afferents (e.g., in a dark environment), causing exacerbated postural and gait instability symptoms.

The main characteristic symptom of BVP is postural and gait instability when walking or standing, while sitting and lying in static conditions are usually not symptomatic. Another common characteristic symptom of BVP is oscillopsia, which occurs when the patient's head and body move actively (e.g., walking as well as rapid head-turning from side to side) or passively (e.g., riding in a car), and is characterized by blurred vision. In addition, some patients often present with chronic dizziness, recurrent vertigo, deafness, and tinnitus. Most patients with BVP present with insidious initial symptoms, and because the disease progresses slowly and progressively, most patients have significant vestibular impairment at the time of presentation. The cochlear and vestibular nerves may be involved simultaneously or sequentially during the course of the disease, and vestibular dysfunction may progress acutely or chronically, completely or incompletely, symmetrically or asymmetrically, and with or without hearing loss. Bedside examinations in patients with BVP may show a positive Romberg test, bilateral positive vHIT, and dynamic visual acuity loss. Ancillary tests, including vHIT, caloric test, and rotational test, are important in making a definitive diagnosis. The diagnosis of BVP requires a combination of patient history, clinical symptoms, and ancillary findings and needs to be differentiated from other vestibular and non-vestibular disorders that present with postural and gait instability and/or oscillopsia symptoms.

The main treatment for BVP is vestibular rehabilitation. Since the patient's bilateral vestibular function is severely impaired, she cannot maintain her balance function through the VOR or vestibulospinal reflex pathways. The main compensatory mechanism is sensory replacement, in which the lost bilateral vestibular functions are replaced through visual, proprioceptive, and cervico-ocular reflex pathways. The relevant education to patients is also of great importance for the treatment and rehabilitation of patients.

## Bibliography

Strupp M, Kim JS, Murofushi T, et al. Bilateral vestibulopathy: diagnostic criteria consensus document of the Classification Committee of the Bárány Society. J Vestib Res. 2017;27(4):177–89.

Wang E, Shan X. Bilateral vestibular disease. Beijing Med. 2018;40(8):733–7.

Ward BK, Tarnutzer AA. Editorial: bilateral vestibulopathy-current knowledge and future directions to improve its diagnosis and treatment. Front Neurol. 2018;9:762.

# Vestibular Paroxysmia

# 10

Haijin Yi

## 10.1 Summary of Medical Records

Patient, female, 70 years old. Complaint: recurrent vertigo attacks with left tinnitus for more than 5 years, aggravated for 20 days. Present history: In 2013, the patient had her first episode of vertigo, which lasted for about a few seconds. The vertigo was a feeling of dizziness and imbalance, with no significant rotation sensation, and was accompanied by tinnitus, but without significant hearing loss or headache. She had several similar episodes of vertigo and tinnitus symptoms and was treated for Meniere disease, but the treatment was not effective. For the past year, the episodes of vertigo have recurred on average once every half a month, with tinnitus at a high pitch, and the episodes of these symptoms were intermittent and each attack lasted for a few seconds, with intermittent attacks. In the past 20 days, the vertigo attacks of the patient were frequent, the symptoms worsened, the tinnitus persisted, and was accompanied by headache symptoms, and she was seen on May 29, 2018. Examination: no abnormalities in both external auditory canals and tympanic membranes, and negative for Romberg test, Fukuda stepping test, Babinski-Weil gait test, head impulse test, Dix-Hallpike test, and roll test. Pure tone audiometry: normal hearing in the right ear, and mild hearing loss in the left ear, with mean hearing threshold of approximately 25 dBHL for air conduction and 20 dBHL for bone conduction. Tympanometry: type A tympanograms. Otoacoustic emission: normal in the right ear, and not elicited at all frequencies in the left ear. Electrocochleography: left ear–SP/AP = 0.51. Electronystagmography: negative spontaneous nystagmus and head shaking nystagmus, normal saccade test, normal smooth pursuit test (type II), normal optokinetic nystagmus. Caloric test: hypofunction of the left horizontal semicircular canal, with directional preponderance (DP) = 35%. Enhanced MRI of the internal auditory meatus showed the cross-compression of the left posterior inferior cerebellar artery and the eighth cranial nerve (Fig. 10.1). Diagnosis of vestibular paroxysmia was made. Treatment: oral flunarizine hydrochloride 5 mg once at night for 2 weeks and oral carbamazepine 100 mg once a day, increasing to 200 mg once a day after 3 days. The patient's symptoms resolved significantly after 2 weeks of treatment. The patient discontinued using carbamazepine due to the drug's adverse effects such as nausea and vomiting associated with it and had difficulty in adhering to the continued use of the drug. After discontinuation of the drug, vertigo and tinnitus occasionally occurred, but the degree of symptoms was less than before.

H. Yi (✉)
Department of Otolaryngology, Head and Neck Surgery, Beijing Tsinghua Changgung Hospital, Tsinghua University, Beijing, China

© Scientific and Technical Documentation Press 2023

X. Shan, E. Wang (eds.), *Interpretation of Vertigo Cases*, Experts' Perspectives on Medical Advances, https://doi.org/10.1007/978-981-99-6995-1_10

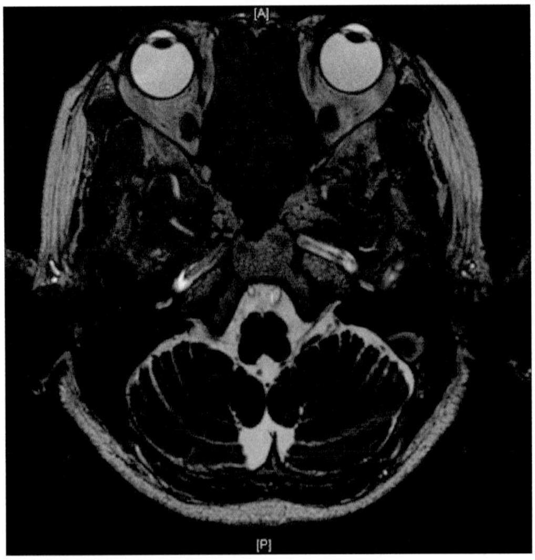


**Fig. 10.1** Enhanced brain MRI at the internal auditory meatus level. Showing the neurovascular cross-compression of the left eighth cranial nerve and the left posterior inferior cerebellar artery

## 10.2 Case Study

The patient was an elderly female with a history of recurrent vertigo attacks with left tinnitus for more than 5 years. Her episodes of vertigo were frequent, each lasting only a few seconds, and mostly accompanied by tinnitus. The otologic examination showed no abnormal findings. The Romberg's test, the Fukuda stepping test, the Babinski-Weil gait test, and head impulse test, the Dix-Hallpike test, and roll test were negative. Pure tone audiometry showed a mean hearing threshold of 25 dBHL for the left air conduction. The otoacoustic emission of the left ear was not elicited. Electrocochleography showed the left ear-SP/AP ratio was 0.51. Spontaneous nystagmus and head-shaking nystagmus were negative, saccade test and smooth pursuit test were normal, optokinetic nystagmus was normal, but caloric test showed reduced left horizontal semicircular canal function with directional preponderance (DP) = 35%. Enhanced MRI of the internal auditory meatus showed the cross-compression of the left posterior inferior cerebellar artery and the eighth cranial nerve. Based on the history, clinical presentation, and examination findings, the patient was diagnosed with vestibular paroxysmia and was treated with appropriate medications. The diagnosis of vestibular paroxysmia was further supported by the effective treatment with oral carbamazepine. The patient's symptoms were significantly relieved after 2 weeks of drug treatment, but she had difficulty in continuing to the use of carbamazepine because of reaction to the drug. The patient experienced significant nausea and vomiting with oral carbamazepine and she had occasional episodes of vertigo and tinnitus after stopping the drug, but the degree of symptoms was less than before.

## 10.3 Case Review

Vestibular paroxysmia is a vestibular disorder that manifests primarily as recurrent transient episodes of vertigo and balance disturbances with or without hearing loss, and may also be associated with tinnitus symptoms. The etiology and pathogenesis of the disease are not well understood. Some studies have suggested that neurovascular cross-compression is the cause of transient vertigo attacks in vestibular paroxysmia. Some scholars have proposed a peripheral hypothesis for the pathogenesis of vestibular paroxysmia, considering that the pathogenesis of vestibular paroxysmia is similar to that of trigeminal neuralgia, which is caused by the compression of nerves by blood vessels, resulting in local nerve demyelination, ectopic impulses, short circuit or pseudosynaptic formation between adjacent nerve fibers, causing the excessive transmission of action potentials between adjacent nerves and the excessive release of nerve impulses, and then causing vertigo symptoms. Other scholars have proposed a central hypothesis for the pathogenesis of vestibular paroxysmia, considering that contact between vessels and nerves causes significant clinical symptoms only when the contact occurs at the cranial nerve roots into the brainstem region, but many scholars have found that approximately 70% of individuals with close contact between the trigeminal nerve or facial nerve and vessels were asymptomatic.

The Barany Society issued diagnostic criteria for vestibular paroxysmia in 2016, and a diagnosis of definite vestibular paroxysmia requires each of the following criteria: (1) at least 10 episodes of spontaneous rotational or non-rotational vertigo; (2) episode duration of less than 1 min; (3) stereotyped symptoms in some patients; (4) response to a treatment with carbamazepine or oxcarbazepine; and (5) not better explained by another diagnosis. The diagnosis of probable vestibular paroxysmia requires each of the following criteria: (a) at least five episodes of rotational or non-rotational vertigo; (b) episode duration less than 5 min; (c) vertigo onset as spontaneous or induced by certain head movements; (d) stereotyped symptoms in some patients; and (e) not better explained by other diagnoses. The main differences between the diagnostic criteria of definite vestibular paroxysmia and probable vestibular paroxysmia are as follows. (1) Number of vertigo episodes: at least ten episodes in definite vestibular paroxysmia, while five or more episodes in probable vestibular paroxysmia. (2) Vertigo attacks are spontaneous in definite vestibular paroxysmia, but in probable vestibular paroxysmia, vertigo attacks can be spontaneous or induced by head movements such as left or right head turning. (3) Duration of vertigo episodes: vertigo episodes shorter than 1 min in definite vestibular paroxysmia and within 5 min in probable vestibular paroxysmia. Medications such as carbamazepine (200–800 mg daily) or oxcarbazepine (300–900 mg daily) are usually effective for vestibular paroxysmia, and a positive response to the drugs further supports the diagnosis. Further research is needed to determine the precise drug dose used for diagnosis and treatment of vestibular paroxysmia. A study including 32 patients showed a 10% reduction in the frequency of vertigo episodes, with the reduced intensity and duration of symptoms in vestibular paroxysmia after treatments with these drugs. For patients who cannot tolerate these drugs, other sodium channel blockers, such as phenytoin sodium or sodium valproate, may be alternatives; however, there are no available studies on the efficacy of phenytoin sodium or sodium valproate for vestibular paroxysmia. Although some reports suggest that some patients with vestibular paroxysmia have been successfully treated surgically, the choice of decompression surgery should be made with caution because of the risk of intraoperative or postoperative vasospasm leading to brainstem infarction. Surgical treatment is only indicated for patients who cannot tolerate the medications.

## Bibliography

Brandt T, Strupp M, Dieterich M. Vestibular paroxysmia: a treatable neurovascular cross-compression syndrome. J Neurol. 2016;263 Suppl 1:S90–6.

Donahue JH, Ornan DA, Mukherjee S. Imaging of vascular compression syndromes. Radiol Clin N Am. 2017;55(1):123–38.

Strupp M, Lopez-Escamez JA, Kim JS, et al. Vestibular paroxysmia: diagnostic criteria. J Vestib Res. 2016;26(5-6):409–15.

Ward BK, Gold DR. Tinnitus, oscillopsia, and hyperventilation-induced nystagmus: vestibular paroxysmia. Open J Clin Med Case Rep. 2016;2(7):1100.

# Middle Ear Cholesteatoma with Labyrinthine Fistula

11

Haijin Yi

## 11.1 Summary of Medical Records

Patient, male, 58 years old. Complaint: Hearing loss in the right ear for more than 50 years, recurrent otorrhea in the right ear for more than 7 years, vertigo for 10 days. Present history: The patient had hearing loss in his right ear when he was a child and was not treated. Seven years ago, he developed otorrhea in his right ear without any obvious cause, with further worsened hearing loss in his right ear. Ten days ago, the patient developed vertigo with no obvious cause, with a sense of rotation, right ear pain and headache, and also had fever with a temperature of 38.5 °C. In a local hospital, the patient was diagnosed as chronic middle ear mastoiditis on the right side and suspected having middle ear cholesteatoma. He was treated with intravenous anti-infective medication. Physical examination: The right external auditory canal was congested and swollen, with pus and blood secretions blocking the external auditory canal, and the tympanic membrane was not detected. The Dix-Hallpike test and the roll test were negative. The Romberg test, the Fukuda stepping test, the Babinski-Weil gait test, and the head impulse test were also negative. Pure tone audiometry: complete deafness in the right ear and normal hearing in the left ear. Auditory brainstem response (ABR): the reflex threshold was normal in the left ear and no response was elicited in the right ear at 95 dBHL. Caloric test could not be performed due to acute inflammation in the right ear. Cranial MRI and thin section scan of the internal auditory meatus: the right horizontal semicircular canal was incomplete, the cochlea and the anterior and posterior semicircular canals showed the reduced signals, and mixed signals were seen in the right mastoid air cells and tympanic cavity with irregular surrounding bone. Imaging diagnosis: right middle ear mastoiditis, probable cholesteatomatous lesion involving the inner ear. CT of the temporal bone: the right mastoid air cells were diploeic type, the image of soft tissue density was seen in the right tympanic cavity, mastoid and external auditory canal, localized bone resorption and destruction of the tympanic tegmen, poor morphology of the ossicles with bone resorption, and bone discontinuity in the right horizontal semicircular canal (Fig. 11.1). The clinical diagnosis was right middle ear cholesteatoma and labyrinthine fistula (limited labyrinthitis). Treatment: After preoperative examination and preparation, microscopic combined endoscopic right mastoid radical surgery, and tympanoplasty were performed under general anesthesia. Intraoperatively, purulent discharge in the right external auditory canal was seen, and after cleaning, a reddish inflammatory neoplasm was found and removed. After mastoid opening, a large

H. Yi (✉)
Department of Otolaryngology, Head and Neck Surgery, Beijing Tsinghua Changgung Hospital, Tsinghua University, Beijing, China

© Scientific and Technical Documentation Press 2023

X. Shan, E. Wang (eds.), *Interpretation of Vertigo Cases*, Experts' Perspectives on Medical Advances, https://doi.org/10.1007/978-981-99-6995-1_11

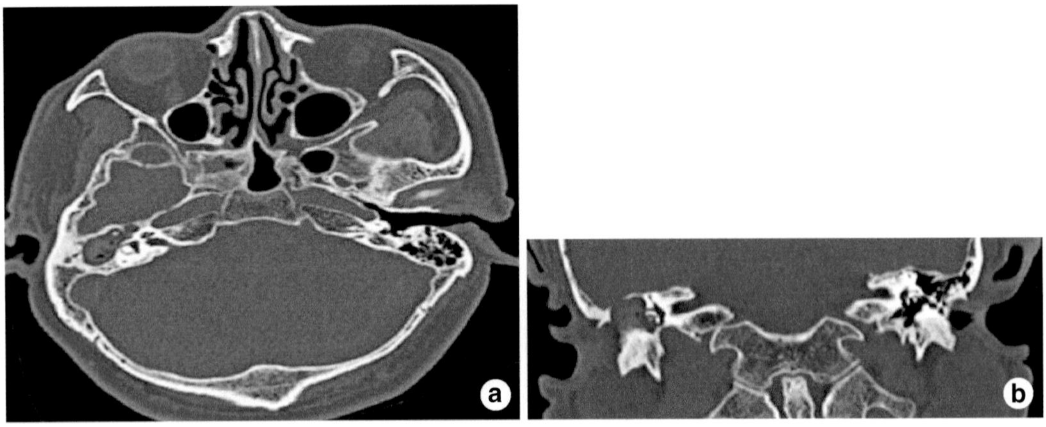


**Fig. 11.1** CT of the temporal bone. (**a**) Axial position; (**b**) coronal position

amount of caseous substance was seen in the mastoid and tympanic cavity, with a bone defect in the tympanic tegmen, and the exposed dura. It was found that the incus was absent, the malleus was partially destroyed, the footplate was incomplete, and the fistula in the horizontal semicircular canal, about 2 mm × 2 mm in size. The residual cholesteatoma lesions on the surface of the fistula were cleared, no exolymphatic fluid leakage was seen, and then the fistula was covered by a small muscle tissue. The osseous canal of the facial nerve in the tympanic segment was absent, the nerve was exposed, and the superficial granulomatous tissues on the nerve were cleared. There was a perforation in the flaccid part of the tympanic membrane. The lesions in the tympanic tegmen and the pyramidal segment of the facial nerve were cleared endoscopically, the tympanic cavity and eustachian tube were closed with muscle and bone wax, the tympanic cavity and mastoid cavity were lined with tragus cartilage and temporalis fascia, and the auricular cavity was shaped. The operative cavity was filled with antibiotic and dexamethasone-soaked gelatin sponge and hemostatic material, and the external ear canal was filled with iodoform gauze. The procedure was completed with intermittent suturing of the subcutaneous and skin incisions and local pressure dressing. The patient was treated postoperatively with intravenous moxifloxacin hydrochloride antibiotic and discharged clinically cured. At postoperative follow-up, the patient had relief of vertigo and headache, no ear drainage, and no change in hearing.

## 11.2 Case Study

The patient was diagnosed with otitis media and treated with ear drops at the local hospital. Since then, he had recurrent symptoms of otorrhea in the right ear, and in the past 7 years, the symptoms of otorrhea in the right ear had worsened. For the recent 10 days, the patient presented with vertigo attacks with right ear pain, headache, and fever. In the local hospital, he was diagnosed with chronic purulent middle ear mastoiditis and suspected with middle ear cholesteatoma, and treated with intravenous antibiotics. On examination in our clinic, the right external auditory canal was found to be congested and swollen with purulent discharge, showing middle ear infection, and also the patient presented with horizontal rightward spontaneous nystagmus. CT of the temporal bone showed soft tissue lesions in the right tympanic cavity, mastoid and external auditory canal, with localized bone resorption and destruction of the tympanic tegmen, poor morphology of the ossicles with bone resorption, and bone discontinuity in the right horizontal semicircular canal (Fig. 11.1). In combination with the patient's history, clinical presentation, and imaging features, the clinical diagnosis of right middle ear cholesteatoma and labyrinthine fistula (limited labyrinthitis) was made despite his negative fistula test. Thus, the patient received surgical treatment. Intraoperatively, as expected, a large number of cholesteatoma-like lesions were seen in the mastoid and tympanic cavity, with extensive destruction of the surrounding tissue structures, leading bone defects in the tympanic tegmen, exposed dura, absent of the incus, partial destruction of the malleus, incomplete structures on the footplate, etc. A fistula of 2 mm × 2 mm in size was seen in the horizontal semicircular canal, and the preoperative clinical diagnosis of the right middle ear cholesteatoma with labyrinthine fistula was confirmed. The patient was clinically cured with surgical treatment as well as postoperative anti-infection treatment. Postoperative follow-up showed that the patient's vertigo and headache were resolved, and he also did not have any further symptoms of ear discharge.

## 11.3 Case Review

Labyrinthine fistula, also known as limited labyrinthitis, is one of the common complications of middle ear cholesteatoma, which is usually caused by cholesteatoma invading the labyrinthine bone. Cholesteatoma destroys bone structures primarily by both local compression due to the distending growth of cholesteatoma and chemical erosion of the bone. The cholesteatoma stroma has high collagenase activity, which can cause cleavage of collagen molecules within the bone tissue, resulting in erosive destruction of the surrounding bone tissue. Studies have shown that 5% to 20% of patients with middle ear cholesteatoma have an associated labyrinthine fistula, and more than 90% of labyrinthine fistulas are located in the horizontal semicircular canal. And other structures, such as the superior semicircular canal, the posterior semicircular canal, the tympanic promontory, the oval window, the cochlea, and the internal auditory meatus, may also be destroyed. The horizontal semicircular canal and facial nerve canal are often involved at the same time because of their anatomical proximity. Patients may present with typical clinical symptoms, including vertigo, but some patients do not present with bone-conducted hearing loss even after occurring of perilymphatic fistula. The development of imaging techniques has improved the preoperative diagnosis of labyrinthine fistula, and imaging examination can be used for intraoperative determination of fistula size and location. However, the preoperative confirmation of labyrinthine fistula remains relatively difficult. For the preoperative diagnosis of labyrinthine fistula, patient's vestibular symptoms, fistula test, and imaging are not sufficient indicators for the definitive diagnosis of labyrinthine fistula, and the absence of vertigo symptoms or a negative fistula test do not exclude the presence of labyrinthine fistula. It was reported that the positive rate for fistula tests was from 24% to 72%, and a negative fistula test can be caused by cholesteatoma tissue obstructing around the fistula during the fistula test, resulting in a low diagnostic accuracy of the test. The reported positive rates of preoperative temporal bone CT scan for the diagnosis of labyrinthine fistula were various, with a positive rate of 93% to 97% and a false-positive rate of no more than 5% for high-resolution CT. The confirmatory method for the diagnosis of labyrinthine fistula is what is seen on intraoperative exploration.

The management of the labyrinthine fistula depends on the size and location of the fistula, the nature of the lesion, and the patient's specific situation. Labyrinthine fistulas are classified mostly according to Dornhoffer's criteria: type I fistula, in which there is the limited destruction of the bony labyrinth and the endosteum is intact; type II fistula, in which the lesion breaks through the endosteum and opens the perilymphatic space; and type III fistula, in which the perilymphatic space opens and the membranous labyrinth is involved. Although in type I and II fistulas, cholesteatoma tissue does not directly penetrate the membranous labyrinth, stimulation of the membranous labyrinth due to the specific chemical effect and the pressure action of cholesteatoma tissue and the long-term infection of the middle ear cavity acting on the broken labyrinth can penetrate the intact membranous labyrinth into the perilymphatic fluid, resulting in bone-conduction hearing loss in some patients. Type III fistula shows the involvement of both the bony and membranous labyrinths, with the fistula communicating with the membranous labyrinth to form a dead labyrinth. 73.7% of patients with labyrinthine fistulas also have combined bone destruction in the bony canal of the facial nerve, the tegmen of the antrum, and part of the anterior wall of the sigmoid sinus. Bone destructions in these structures indicate that the cholesteatoma is highly aggressive and there is possibly the destruction of the labyrinthine bone; therefore, if bone destruction is found intraoperatively in these sites, care should be taken when clearing the lesions semicircular canal or the tympanic capsule area because of the possible presence of labyrinthine fistula.

The managements of labyrinthine fistulas are controversial. Some scholars believe that intraoperative harassment of the fistula may lead to further hearing loss, so careful protection of the fistula during mastoid surgery may preserve or improve some hearing postoperatively. However, some scholars believe that leaving over the cholesteatoma stroma may result in long-term postoperative otorrhea, while removal of the cholesteatoma stroma may prevent toxic changes in the cochlea. Careful removing of the surface lesion of the fistula during surgery and rapid closure of the fistula with a graft may serve to protect vestibular and cochlear functions. The complete removal of the cholesteatoma stroma and the repair of the fistula depend on the doctor's experiences and skills as a surgeon. Care and caution are required when separating the cholesteatoma stroma from the fistula surface, and then the fistula should be repaired with prepared repair material as quickly as possible. The repair materials include temporalis fascia or muscle, bone coat, cartilage, or bone powder in the case of type III fistulas with canal occlusion. In middle ear cholesteatoma, the possibility of a labyrinthine fistula is considered in any intraoperative management of the lesion, and intraoperative exploration is a reliable method of diagnosing a labyrinthine fistula. In addition, in the presence of labyrinthine fistula, the facial nerve canal should also be checked. In the management of the labyrinthine fistula, the choice should be individualized according to the patient's condition, and the cholesteatoma stroma should be removed as much as possible to reduce the possibility of recurrence and the fistula should be repaired promptly, but there is a risk of bone conduction hearing impairment during the removal of the cholesteatoma stroma from the fistula surface, so the cleaning process should be performed carefully to preserve the labyrinth function as much as possible.

## Bibliography

Geerse S, de Wolf MJF, Ebbens FA, van Spronsen E. Management of labyrinthine fistula: hearing preservation versus prevention of residual disease. Eur Arch Otorhinolaryngol. 2017;274(10):3605–12.

Lim J, Gangal A, Gluth MB. Surgery for cholesteatomatous labyrinthine fistula. Ann Otol Rhinol Laryngol. 2017;126(3):205–15.

Meyer A, Bouchetemblé P, Costentin B, et al. Lateral semicircular canal fistula in cholesteatoma: diagnosis and management. Eur Arch Otorhinolaryngol. 2016;273(8):2055–63.

# 12 Light Cupula

Hui Leng

## 12.1 Summary of Medical Records

Patient, female, 32 years old. Complaint: Recurrent episodes of positional vertigo for 3 days. Present history: The patient had symptoms of vertigo with the changes of head positions 3 days ago, visual rotation with nausea and vomiting, no hearing loss, tinnitus, and ear fullness, and also no headache, and at a local hospital she was diagnosed with benign paroxysmal positional vertigo (BPPV), which was not resolved by particle repositioning maneuver. And then the patient visited our clinic on May 18, 2017. Past history: no previous history of vertigo, no history of migraine, denied history of chronic diseases such as hypertension and diabetes mellitus. Examination: general condition was good, and there were no abnormal signs on general examination and neurological examination. Otologic examination: no abnormalities in the external auditory canal and tympanic membrane. Pure tone audiometry: normal hearing in both ears. Saccade test: normal. Smooth pursuit test: Type I. Optokinetic test: normal. Caloric test: normal vestibular responses bilaterally. Video head impulse test (v-HIT): negative. Positional tests: bilateral Dix-Hallpike tests were negative; bow and lean test and multipositional roll tests: showing "zero plane" and persistent direction-changing positional nystagmus (DCPN) (Table 12.1). Diagnosis: light cupula of the left horizontal semicircular canal. Treatment: flunarizine 10 mg once a night for 1 week. Follow-up: After 1 week, the symptoms of positional vertigo and nystagmus disappeared.

H. Leng (✉)
Department of Otolaryngology, Affiliated Hospital of Liaoning Traditional Chinese Medicine University, Shenyang, China

© Scientific and Technical Documentation Press 2023

X. Shan, E. Wang (eds.), *Interpretation of Vertigo Cases*, Experts' Perspectives on Medical Advances, https://doi.org/10.1007/978-981-99-6995-1_12

**Table 12.1** Results of sitting head bow and lean test and multipositional supine roll test

| Head position | Nystagmus | Direction of nystagmus | Slowphase velocity (°/s) | Duration of nystagmus (min) | Zero plane |
|---|---|---|---|---|---|
| Upright in sitting | + | ← | 1.3 | >1 | |
| Sitting with head down 30° | – | | | | 1st zero plane |
| Supine position | + | ← | 4.6 | >1 | |
| Supine with head turning 15° to the left | – | | | | 2nd zero plane |
| Supine with head turning 30° to the left | + | → | 4.9 | >1 | |
| Supine with head turning 45° to the left | + | → | 5.2 | >1 | |
| Left lateral recumbent position | + | → | 7.3 | >1 | |
| Prone position | + | → | 3.7 | >1 | |
| Prone with head turning 15° to the left | – | | | | 3rd zero plane |
| Prone with head turning 30° to the left | – | | | | |
| Prone with head turning 45° to the left | + | ← | 3.5 | >1 | |
| Right lateral recumbent position | + | ← | 8.7 | >1 | |
| Supine position | + | ← | 3.6 | >1 | |

## 12.2 Case Study

The patient is a young woman who complained of recurrent episodes of positional vertigo for 3 days without the symptoms of hearing loss, tinnitus, or ear fullness, and also no migraine symptoms. She had no clear cause for her vertigo and no previous history of vertigo. At the local hospital, the patient was diagnosed as BPPV and treated with the particle repositioning maneuver, but with no efficacy. The audiological examination showed normal hearing. Saccade test, smooth pursuit test, optokinetic test, caloric test and v-HIT were all negative, but the sitting head bow and lean test and multipositional roll test showed the presence of multiple "zero planes," and the roll test could induce persistent geotropic DCPN. The patient had symptoms and nystagmus characteristics for light cupula of the horizontal semicircular canal and met the diagnostic criteria of light cupula, and the treatment with particle repositioning maneuver was ineffective for the patient. Patients with light cupula disease usually complain of recurrent episodes of positional vertigo or dizziness, which may occur when lowering or raising the head, lying down, sitting up, or turning from side to side, with long duration and variable frequency of episodes. Nystagmus in light cupula disease has the following characteristics. (1) Sitting head bow and lean test and supine roll test induce persistent geotropic DCPN with no latency period and a duration of more than 1 min. (2) The presence of the zero plane, i.e., a plane in which nystagmus disappears during slow rotation of the head to the left or right in the supine position. (3) The presence of horizontal nystagmus toward the healthy side in the supine position, and horizontal nystagmus toward the affected side in the prone position. (4) Nystagmus is mostly absent in the upright head position. (5) Nystagmus component is predominantly horizontal, with a vertical or torsional component in 40–80% of cases. (6) Intensity of nystagmus: 90° position vertical to zero plane > prone position > supine position > sit-to-stand position. Currently, the main diagnostic criteria for light cupula are as follows: persistent geotropic DCPN on the roll test, with no significant latency and fatigability; the presence of a zero plane on the roll test, i.e., no nystagmus present when rolled to the plane, and the zero plane usually appears in the supine position with the head turning 15°–30° to the affected side; ineffective treatment with repeated repositioning maneuvers based on the horizontal semicircular canal BPPV; and spontaneous healing after 1–4 weeks. In addition, the symptoms and nystagmus in the light cupula are quite similar to those in the canalithiasis of horizontal semicircular canal, so they need to be differentiated. The latter can also show geotropic DCPN on the roll test, but the nystagmus lasts less than 1 min, usually with a latency period and fatigability, and is usually effective with repositioning treatment.

## 12.3 Case Review

The light cupula theory was first proposed in 1956 by Aschan et al. They observed that persistent geotropic nystagmus could occur after drinking alcohol and thus this nystagmus was called as alcoholic positional nystagmus, suggesting that the mechanism of alcoholic positional nystagmus is that because the cupula is closer to the capillaries, alcohol diffuses into the cupula faster than into the nearby endolymphatic fluid, causing the decrease of cupula mass relative to the endolymph, i.e., forming a light cupula. In certain head position, the light cupula is subjected to sustained upward buoyancy, with deflection to the side of the utricle. In 2002, Shigeno described light cupula nystagmus and its characteristics: persistent DCPN. In 2004, Hiruma et al. clinically encountered patients with light cupula showing the nystagmus similar to alcoholic positional nystagmus. In 2014 and 2016, Kim and Ichijo et al., respectively, reported the nystagmus characteristics and zero-plane phenomenon of light cupula, and the disease is gradually recognized and understood.

A better understanding of the concept of zero plane is required for the recognition and study of light cupula disease. The definition of zero plane: the position plane where persistent DCPN disappears during the patient's head position changes. Mechanism of zero-plane production: the long axis of the cupula in this plane is parallel to the line of gravity and thus the cupula does not oscillate. The first zero plane: The positional plane in which the patient is seated and their positional nystagmus disappears with gentle forward or backward flexion of the head. The second zero plane: The patient is in the supine position and when the positional nystagmus disappears with the slow lateral rotation of the head to the right or left, often at 15°–30° of lateral rotation, this position plane is the second zero plane. The third zero plane: The position plane where the positional nystagmus disappears again with the slow lateral turn of the patient's head to the right or left in the prone position. The mechanism of light cupula disease is not well understood and the following hypotheses exist. (1) Decreased density of the cupula. (2) An increase in endolymphatic specific gravity, leading to a relative decrease in the mass of the cupula. (3) Light cupula due to the adhesion of the decalcified degenerate light otolith particles or floating cells in endolymphatic fluid to the cupula. (4) As a result of a morphologic change in the cupula.

Light cupula disease is easily misdiagnosed as BPPV and can account for 4.9% of patients diagnosed as BPPV, 9.4% of patients presenting with horizontal DCPN, and 14.2% of patients presenting with geotropic horizontal DCPN. Among the patients with the light cupula, women are significantly more than men, with a ratio of 2:1 or 3:1. About 70% of patients with the light cupula had previous history of episodic vertigo, 30–50% had history of BPPV, 40% had history of migraine, 10% complained of ipsilateral hearing loss, and some patients had Meniere disease-like episodes. Repositioning maneuvers such as barbecue maneuver used for the treatments of BPPV are ineffective for the light cupula. Medications such as flunarizine and vestibular rehabilitation are helpful in the control and relief of vertigo, autonomic symptoms, and psychological condition of patients. The prognosis of the disease is good.

## Bibliography

Ichijo H. Neutral position of persistent direction-changing positional nystagmus. Eur Arch Otorhinolaryngol. 2016;273(2):311–6.

Imai T, Matsuda K, Takeda N, et al. Light cupula: the pathophysiological basis of persistent geotropic positional nystagmus. BMJ Open. 2015;5(1):e006607.

Kim MB, Hong SM, Choi H, et al. The light cupula: an emerging new concept for positional vertigo. J Audiol Otol. 2018;22(1):1–5.

# Part II

# Central Vertigo Disorders

# 13 Central Positional Vertigo Due to Non-Hodgkin's Lymphoma of the Fourth Ventricle of the Cerebellum

Hui Leng

## 13.1 Summary of Medical Records

Patient, male, 60 years old. Complaint: Recurrent episodes of dizziness and positional vertigo for 3 months. Present history: The patient developed dizziness 3 months ago with no obvious cause, and dizziness occurred when he changed his head position, with a sensation of rotating vision and nausea and vomiting, without obvious tinnitus and hearing loss. He had been diagnosed with "benign paroxysmal positional vertigo (BPPV)" at a hospital and was given several repositioning maneuvers, but did not receive treatment efficacy. On November 25, 2016, the patient came to our hospital and was admitted for further diagnosis and treatment. The patient had no history of fever, ear pain, or ear discharge since the onset of the disease. Past history: no history of chronic ear disease, migraine, surgical trauma, ototoxic drug application. He had no family history of hereditary disease. On admission: temperature 36.5 °C, pulse 56/min, respiration 18/min, blood pressure 125/85 mm Hg. No abnormal findings on general and otologic examinations. Auxiliary examinations were as follows. Audiometry: normal hearing in both ears. Nystagmography: spontaneous nystagmus was negative. The smooth pursuit test was type III curve. Caloric test showed bilateral vestibular hypofunction. Positional tests: the left Dix-Hallpike test induced clockwise torsional nystagmus with no significant latency and nystagmus duration >100 s, the right Dix-Hallpike test was negative, and the roll tests were negative. Brain MRI and enhancement scan (Fig. 13.1): a round-like occupying lesion was seen on the right side of the fourth ventricle, showing an iso-$T_1$ slightly long $T_2$ signal image, measuring about

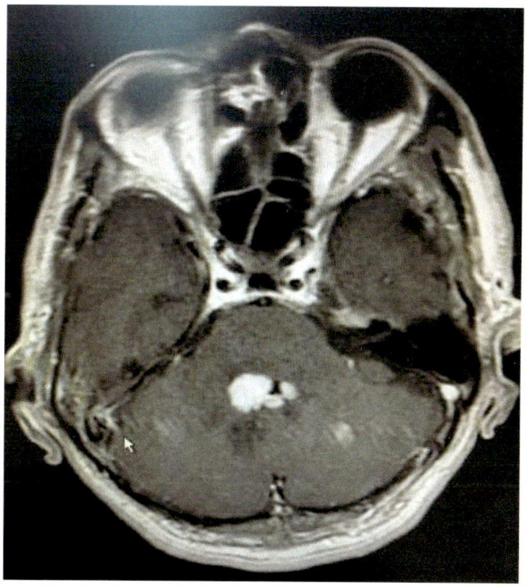

Fig. 13.1 Brain MRI enhancement scan. A tumor of 1.4 cm × 1.1 cm × 1.6 cm showed in the cerebellum (fourth ventricle), with a postoperative pathological diagnosis of non-Hodgkin's lymphoma of the cerebellum (fourth ventricle)

H. Leng (✉)
Department of Otolaryngology, Affiliated Hospital of Liaoning Traditional Chinese Medicine University, Shenyang, China

© Scientific and Technical Documentation Press 2023

X. Shan, E. Wang (eds.), *Interpretation of Vertigo Cases*, Experts' Perspectives on Medical Advances, https://doi.org/10.1007/978-981-99-6995-1_13

1.4 cm × 1.1 cm × 1.6 cm, with the compressed fourth ventricle and the lower part of the midbrain aqueduct, surrounded by lamellar long $T_1$ long and $T_2$ edema signals, involving the right cerebral peduncle. Brain MRI enhancement scan showed the lesion was significantly enhanced, and two small enhancing nodular images were also seen in the fourth ventricle, with a diameter of 4–5 mm. The clinical diagnoses were central paroxysmal positional vertigo (CPPV) and cerebellar (fourth ventricle) tumor. The patient received surgical treatment, and the postoperative pathological diagnosis was non-Hodgkin's lymphoma of the cerebellum (fourth ventricle).

## 13.2 Case Study

The patient was an elderly male who complained of dizziness and recurrent episodes of positional vertigo for 3 months, with nausea and vomiting during the vertigo attacks, but without significant tinnitus and hearing loss. The patient was diagnosed with "BPPV" by a hospital and was treated with particle repositioning maneuvers but the treatments failed. After admission, the patient's smooth pursuit test showed type III curve, and the left Dix-Hallpike test was positive. Based on the patient's history of repeated episodes of positional vertigo and clinical manifestations, he was first considered to have BPPV, because it is the most common clinical disorder of positional vertigo. However, the patient's smooth pursuit test showed type III curve, and although the Dix-Hallpike test on another side was not positive, his positional nystagmus was an atypical nystagmus manifestation of BPPV, showing simple torsional nystagmus without a significant latency period, and the nystagmus lasted more than 100 s. Since the patient was not effectively treated with multiple repositioning maneuvers for BPPV, it was considered that the patient might have central positional vertigo/nystagmus, and he received imaging examination to rule out a central lesion. Brain MRI and enhancement scan showed a tumor-like lesion in the cerebellum (fourth ventricle). The patient was given surgical treatment, and the postoperative pathological diagnosis was non-Hodgkin's lymphoma of the cerebellum (fourth ventricle).

## 13.3 Case Review

Positional vertigo or nystagmus is usually caused by peripheral vestibular disorders, especially BPPV, but some positional vertigo or nystagmus can also be caused by central lesions, i.e., the so-called central positional vertigo or nystagmus. It is important to distinguish quickly and precisely between central and peripheral vertigo or nystagmus. Although central positional vertigo or nystagmus is much less common than BPPV, its episodes, clinical manifestations, and characteristics of the positional test can be very similar to BPPV, so it is important to be alert and differentiate. Central positional vertigo or nystagmus was first described by Riesco-Macllure in 1957 and has since been recognized and must be widely noted by clinicians because it is easily misdiagnosed as BPPV. Common disorders that cause central vertigo or nystagmus include: (1) Brain tumors, such as cerebellar and fourth ventricle tumors, auditory neuroma (vestibular schwannoma) or other cerebellopontine angle tumors. (2) Cerebrovascular disease, such as posterior circulation ischemia, dorsolateral infarction of the fourth ventricle, and cerebellar or brainstem hemorrhage. (3) Other central neuropathies. Detailed examination is needed to diagnose and differentiate patients presenting with positional vertigo or nystagmus in clinical practice to prevent misdiagnosis or missed diagnosis and delayed treatment.

## Bibliography

Brandt T, Dieterich M. The dizzy patient: don't forget disorders of the central vestibular system. Nat Rev Neurol. 2017;13(6):352–62.

Brozovich A, Ewing D, Burns E, et al. Primary CNS lymphoma arising from the 4th ventricle: a case report and review of the literature. Case Rep Oncol Med. 2019;2019:2671794.

Cho BH, Kim SH, Kim SS, et al. Central positional nystagmus associated with cerebellar tumors: clinical and topographical analysis. J Neurol Sci. 2017;373:147–51.

Macdonald NK, Kaski D, Saman Y, et al. Central positional nystagmus: a systematic literature review. Front Neurol. 2017;8:141.

Power L, Murray K, Drummond KJ, et al. Fourth ventricle ependymoma mimicking benign paroxysmal positional vertigo. Neurology. 2018;91(7):327–8.

# Medulloblastoma of the Fourth Ventricle with Positional Vertigo

14

Jinmei Liu

## 14.1 Summary of Medical Records

Patient, female, 29 years old. Complaint: episodes of vertigo for 3 months. Present history: In the past 3 months, the patient had recurrent episodes of vertigo, which were mostly related to the changes of body and head positions and worsened when lying down, but significantly better after turning over. Since the onset of the disease, there was occasional numbness in the right upper limb and lateral pulsion during walking, but there were no symptoms of dyspnea, incontinence, ataxia, limb movement disorders, facial numbness, and consciousness disorders. Past history: having a history of migraine headache with tightness, right-sided, moderate pain, sometimes with nausea, photophobia and phonophobia, with no special treatment for the migraine. No history of hypertension, diabetes mellitus, or heart disease. No history of smoking or alcohol consumption. Her father also had a history of migraine. The patient was admitted to the hospital on September 17, 2015. Physical examination: temperature 35.9 °C, pulse 76 beats/min, respiration 18 breaths/min, and blood pressure 110/78 mmHg. Neurological examination: clear consciousness, fluent speech, normal findings for cranial nerve examination, normal muscle strength and muscle tone of the extremities, bilateral biceps tendon reflexes were normal, Babinski's sign, Kirschner's sign, and Brønsted's sign were negative bilaterally. Romberg test was negative, but tandem Romberg test was positive, leaning to the left. Pure tone audiometry: normal average hearing threshold in both ears. Tympanogram: normal type A curves in two ears. Auditory brainstem evoked potentials (ABR): binaural response thresholds of 30 dBHL, good differentiation of each wave, and normal I-V wave intervals. Electrocochleography: normal in both ears. Optokinetic nystagmus test: no abnormality. Gaze test: negative. Caloric test: CP(R) = 23.7%, indicating reduced right horizontal semicircular canal function. Post-rotational nystagmus: the leftward nystagmus with slow phase velocity of 12.6°/s was triggered by suddenly stopping after sustained clockwise rotation, and the rightward nystagmus with slow phase velocity of 38.1°/s was triggered by suddenly stopping after sustained counterclockwise rotation, CP = 50.1%, suggesting obvious asymmetry of nystagmus triggered by stimulating bilateral horizontal semicircular canals. Positional tests: Dix-Hallpike test and roll test were negative. Balance function examination (posturography): in static posture (eyes open), the center of gravity showed anterior-posterior distribution and the total trajectory length of dynamic rocking was 15.3 cm; in static posture (eyes closed), the center of gravity showed central distribution and the total

J. Liu (✉)
Institute of Vertigo, Third Medical Center, PLA General Hospital, Beijing, China

© Scientific and Technical Documentation Press 2023
X. Shan, E. Wang (eds.), *Interpretation of Vertigo Cases*, Experts' Perspectives on Medical Advances, https://doi.org/10.1007/978-981-99-6995-1_14

trajectory length of dynamic rocking was 19.9 cm; standing on sponge mat (eyes open), the center of gravity showed central distribution and the total trajectory length of dynamic rocking was 14.7 cm; standing on sponge mat (eyes closed), the center of gravity showed anterior-posterior distribution and the total trajectory length of dynamic rocking was 41.5 cm. The visual dysmetria test was normal bilaterally. Smooth pursuit test: type II curve. The blood, urine, and stool examinations, coagulation function tests, and biochemical tests were not abnormal. The patient was initially diagnosed with atypical benign paroxysmal positional vertigo (BPPV) and tried to receive the repositioning treatments, but without significant effectiveness. Since the patient had a family history of migraine and was considered to have vestibular migraine and was treated with improving circulation drugs and calcium channel antagonists, which also had poor effectiveness. Brain MRI: showing the longer $T_1$ and $T_2$ signal image, with clear border, size about 38.2 mm × 23.3 mm × 27.5 mm, accompanied with the compression of anterior brainstem and the slight dilation of the fourth ventricle, supratentorial third ventricle, bilateral lateral ventricles. Brain enhancement MRI: indicating a tumor with rich blood supply in the fourth ventricle, considered as ventricular meningioma (Fig. 14.1). Neurosurgery consultation: surgery was recommended. Momentarily, the patient and her family were unwilling to undergo surgical treatment and discharged from the hospital. The patient was subsequently followed up and later the patient reported that she had undergone the resection of the tumor in the fourth ventricle and postoperative radiation therapy at another hospital, and the postoperative pathological diagnosis was medulloblastoma of the fourth ventricle.

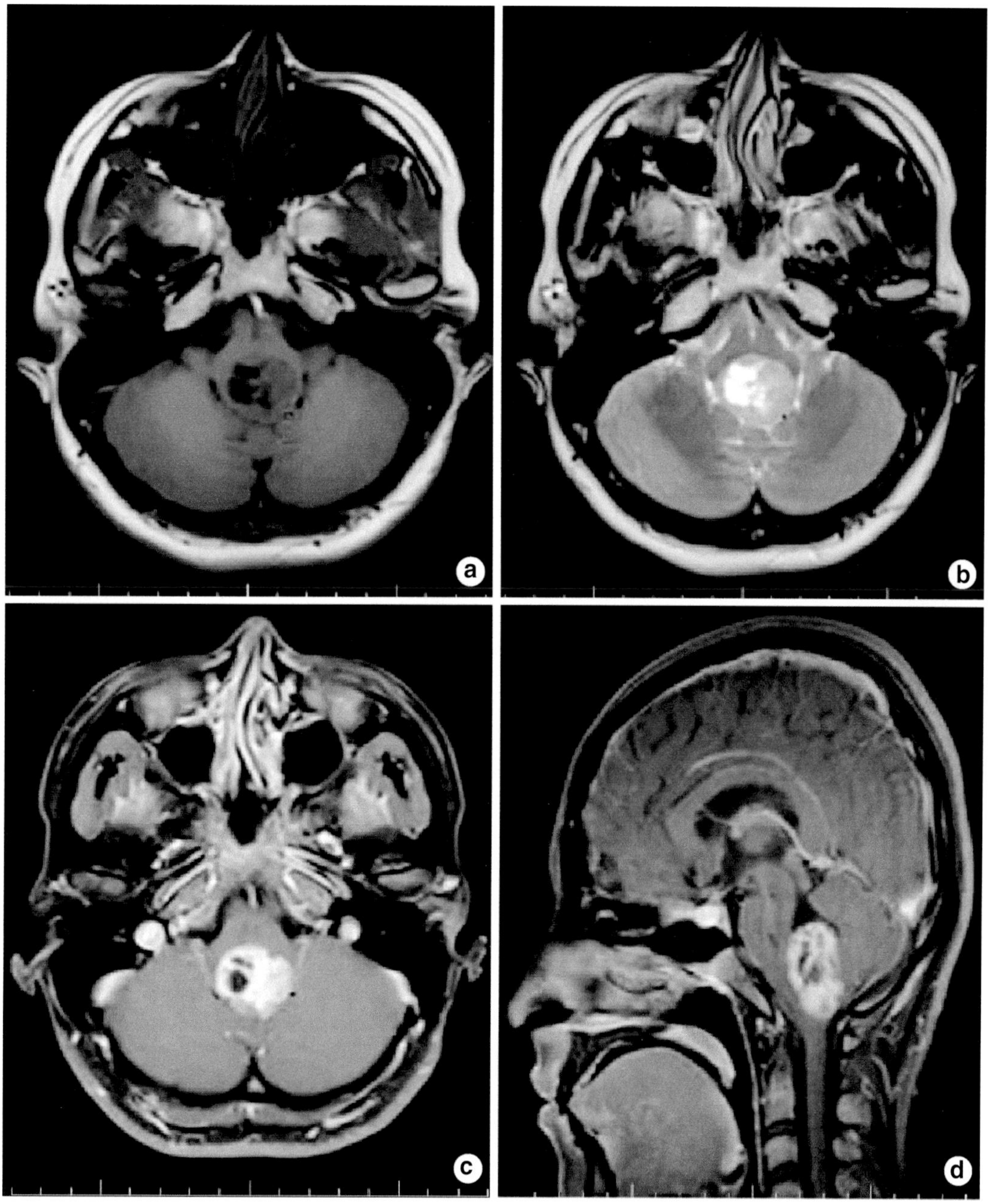


**Fig. 14.1** Brain MRI. Showing an occupying lesion in the fourth ventricle. (**a**) $T_1$WI enhancement; (**b**) $T_2$WI enhancement; (**c**) Axial enhancement; (**d**) Sagittal enhancement. A mass with long $T_1$ and long $T_2$ signals is seen at the base of the fourth ventricle with inhomogeneous signals, within which a strip of tubular flow-void vascular shadow is visible, and the fourth ventricle, medulla oblongata, and adjacent cerebellar hemispheres are significantly compressed, and the lesion is seen to be significantly inhomogeneously enhanced on enhancement scan

## 14.2 Case Study

The patient was a young woman who complained of recurrent vertigo for 3 months. Her vertigo attacks were mostly associated with the changes in body and head positions, feeling symptom worsening when lying down and better after turning over, and the vertigo attacks were accompanied by a sensation of visual spinning that lasted for about a few seconds without nausea or vomiting. The patient's vertigo attacks were characterized by paroxysmal positional vertigo, but were not typical symptoms of BPPV, and the Dix-Hallpike test and roll test were negative, so the patient was initially considered to have atypical BPPV, but treatment with particle repositioning maneuver did not have any significant therapeutic effect. Because the patient had a history of migraine and a family history of migraine, she was considered to have vertiginous migraine attacks, and was given medication for vestibular migraine, but the results were also poor. Since the patient had occasional numbness of the right upper limb and lateral pulsion in walking since the onset of the disease, in order to exclude whether the patient's vertigo symptoms were caused by a central lesion, the patient was given a brain MRI examination on the fourth day after admission, which showed a 38.2 mm × 23.3 mm × 27.5 mm oval occupying lesion in the fourth ventricle with the pressed anterior brainstem and slightly dilated fourth ventricle, the third supratentorial ventricle, and bilateral lateral ventricles. The enhancement brain MRI showed a tumor with rich blood supply in the fourth ventricle, and the diagnosis of ventricular meningioma was considered. The patient was discharged from the hospital and underwent resection of the tumor in the fourth ventricle, with a postoperative pathological diagnosis of medulloblastoma and postoperative radiotherapy in another hospital. Postoperatively, the patient's symptoms of positional vertigo, right upper limb numbness, and lateral pulsion in walking deviation disappeared. The cause for the patient's central positional vertigo and nystagmus was clarified as a medulloblastoma of the fourth ventricle.

## 14.3 Case Review

Positional vertigo is a common symptom, and vertigo attacks caused by changes in head or body positions are often accompanied by positional nystagmus. Positional vertigo is mostly peripheral in nature and is most common in BPPV. Central positional vertigo or nystagmus is sometimes quite similar to BPPV. Central positional nystagmus differs from the nystagmus in BPPV. Central positional nystagmus is commonly without obvious latency period and it is mostly continuous without a tendency to get stronger and to get weaker. Central positional nystagmus commonly presents as vertical positional nystagmus, and sometimes it can be horizontal or torsional nystagmus. The typical clinical manifestations of occupying lesion in the fourth ventricle are the position-induced acute headache, vomiting, vertigo, and disturbance of consciousness, often accompanied by fall attacks and forced head position. Ventricular meningioma and medulloblastoma are more common among the fourth ventricular tumors. Medulloblastoma is the most common fourth ventricular tumor in children and adolescents, and it originates from the cerebellar vermis, rich in vascular tissue, and may be companied with cystic necrosis showing significant enhancement on MRI. Clinicians need to improve their understanding and differentiation of central positional vertigo or nystagmus in the management of positional vertigo or nystagmus, and pay attention to the differentiation from other diseases presenting as positional vertigo or nystagmus, especially BPPV. In patients with atypical vertigo symptoms, uncertainty in the positional test and poor results of repositioning maneuvers, comprehensive physical examination should be performed, supplemented by necessary brain MRI to clarify the diagnosis. This patient was considered to have a central disorder because of atypical positional test findings, positive tendon Romberg test, and left-sided pulsion symptom, and further brain MRI examination enabled a clear diagnosis to be made, allowing the patient to be treated promptly.

## Bibliography

Cho BH, Kim SH, Kim SS, et al. Central positional nystagmus associated with cerebellar tumors: clinical and topographical analysis. J Neurol Sci. 2017;373:147–51.

Macdonald NK, Kaski D, Saman Y, et al. Central positional nystagmus: a systematic literature review. Front Neurol. 2017;8:141.

Power L, Murray K, Drummond KJ, et al. Fourth ventricle ependymoma mimicking benign paroxysmal positional vertigo. Neurology. 2018;91(7):327–8.

# Central Paroxysmal Positional Vertigo Caused by a Cerebellar Tumor

# 15

Hanjun Sun and Qing Sun

## 15.1 Summary of Medical Records

Patient, female, 27 years old. Complaint: Recurrent episodes of position vertigo for more than 2 years. Present history: The patient began to have recurrent episodes of transient vertigo 2 years ago, mostly when getting up or lying down. The vertigo episodes usually lasted for tens of seconds, with a sensation of rotating vision, accompanied by nausea, but without vomiting, no ear symptoms such as tinnitus, ear fullness, and hearing loss, and without the symptoms of headache, convulsions, impaired consciousness, diplopia, choking on water, and dysarthria. The patient had been seen at a local hospital with a positive positional test and was diagnosed with benign paroxysmal positional vertigo (BPPV): canalolithiasis of the left posterior semicircular canal, and was treated with canalith repositioning maneuvers, but there was no improvement in vertigo symptoms. She came to our hospital for further consultation on November 8, 2018. Past history: no history of head trauma, headache, or motion sickness, no family history of motion sickness, headache, or dizziness. Admission examination: general physical examination with no abnormal findings. Otologic examination: no abnormalities in the external auditory canal and tympanic membrane, negative for spontaneous nystagmus. Positional test: lying down test, right roll test, and bilateral Dix-Hallpike test all induced vertical down-beating nystagmus, which had no latency and was paroxysmal in nature, lasting for about 15 s. Although the patient presented with paroxysmal positional vertigo similar to BPPV, her nystagmus characteristics suggested central positional nystagmus. With carefull reading of the patient's original brain MRI performed early on March 10, 2018 at other hospital, a suspicious occupying lesion was indicated in the cerebellar vermis (Fig. 15.1). And then brain MRI enhancement scan was performed, suggesting a suspicious abnormal signal in the cerebellar vermis, and further brain magnetic resonance spectroscopy (MRS) analysis showed elevated Cho and decreased NAA in the focal area of the cerebellar vermis, with imaging features consistent with a low-grade glioma. Four specialists from several well-known hospitals in Beijing consulted with the patient, but the treatment opinions were not consistent. One of them considered that "the cerebellar vermis lesion requires pathological diagnosis, and two options can be taken: first, puncture for pathology; second, as the lesion is not large, it can be removed directly by surgery and diagnosed by pathology after surgery." The second specialist's opinion was "surgery is recommended, and there is no significant impact on life and fertility after surgery." The third specialist did not recommend surgery based

H. Sun · Q. Sun (✉)
Institute of Vertigo, Third Medical Center, PLA General Hospital, Beijing, China

© Scientific and Technical Documentation Press 2023
X. Shan, E. Wang (eds.), *Interpretation of Vertigo Cases*, Experts' Perspectives on Medical Advances, https://doi.org/10.1007/978-981-99-6995-1_15

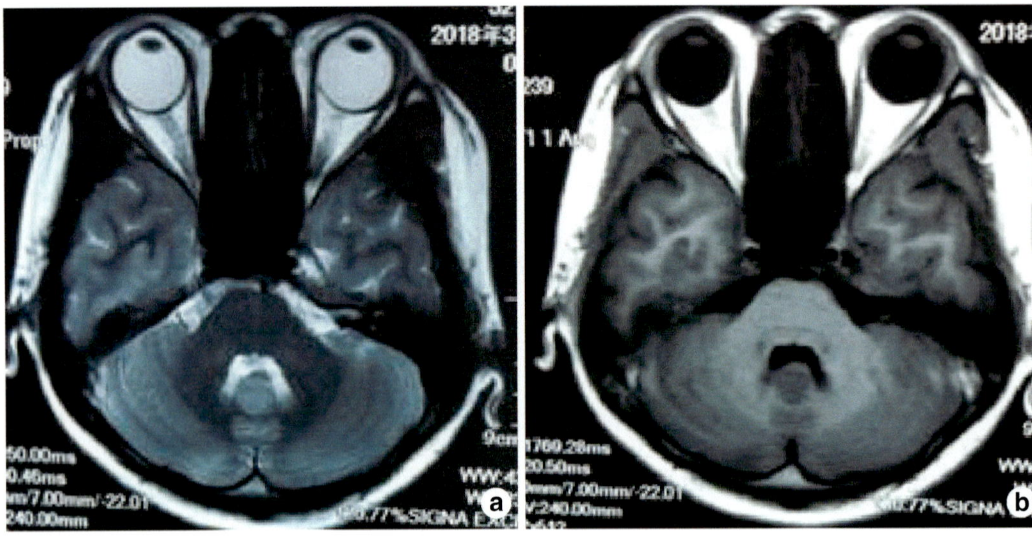


**Fig. 15.1** Brain MRI. (**a**) $T_2$ image; (**b**) $T_2$ Flair image

on the following reasons: firstly, the surgery of cerebellar vermis would aggravate the patient's vertigo symptom, and secondly, the low-grade intracranial tumor might grow faster after surgery. The fourth expert said, "Surgery is not recommended for vertigo caused by cerebellar vermis tumor because (1) The vertigo will worsen after surgery. (2) The lesion area has a role in maintaining balance. (3) The tumor growth is possibly slow and can be followed up". Taking into account the experts' consultation, the patient decided not to receive an operation for the time being, and also not to use the drugs because of the fear of adverse effects. The patient was followed up for 6 months, living a normal working and life with the same vertigo symptoms as before, but with slightly more frequent episodes of vertigo, which may occur every night.

## 15.2 Case Study

The patient was a young woman who complained of recurrent episodes of vertigo for more than 2 years. Her episodes of vertigo were associated with changes in body position, often occurring when she got up or lay down, lasting for a short time of only about tens of seconds. Apart from the symptoms of episodic positional vertigo, the patient presented with no other neurological symptoms. She was diagnosed with benign paroxysmal positional vertigo after a positive positional test at a local hospital, but the patient's vertigo symptoms did not improve with canalith repositioning treatment. The patient's initial diagnosis upon admission was also considered to be BPPV, which is the most common peripheral vestibular disorder and induced by changes in head position relative to the direction of gravity. BPPV presents with recurrent episodes of transient vertigo and characteristic nystagmus, is often self-limiting and prone to recurrence. When presence of typical clinical symptoms, combined with the characteristic nystagmus on positional test, the disease is mostly diagnosed definitively. The typical posterior semicircular canal BPPV mostly shows vertical up-beating nystagmus with torsional component in the Dix-Hallpike test, while the anterior semicircular canal BPPV shows vertical down-beating nystagmus with torsional component in the Dix-Hallpike test or supine straight head-hanging test, or only shows vertical down-beating nystagmus if the torsional nystagmus component is weak. In this case, the patient had negative spontaneous nystagmus, but showed vertical down-beating nystagmus with no latency in several positional tests, such as the lying-down test, the right roll test, and the bilateral Dix-Hallpike tests. With careful reading of the patient's brain MRI performed at other hospital 6 months earlier, an occupying lesion in the cerebellar vermis was indicated. Further brain MRI enhancement and magnetic resonance spectroscopy (MRS) showed a cerebellar vermis lesion with imaging features consistent with a low-grade glioma. The patient was meticulously consulted by four specialists from several well-known hospitals in Beijing, but the treatment opinions were not consistent. A expert believed that "the cerebellar vermis lesion requires pathological diagnosis, two options can be taken, one is to puncture for pathology; another one is direct surgical excision because the lesion is not large, followed by postoperative pathological diagnosis." Another expert "recommends surgery, and considers the patient's postoperative life and fertility may not be affected." The third expert "does not recommend surgery because vertigo will be aggravated after surgery, and low grade intracranial tumor may grow faster after surgery." The fourth expert "does not recommend surgery for the patient with vertigo caused by cerebellar vermis tumor based on following reasons: (1) vertigo will worsen after surgery. (2) The lesion area has a role in maintaining balance. (3) It is possible that the tumor is growing slowly and the patient can be followed up with medication such as clonazepam and topiramate tablets". The patient did not want to undergo surgery after considering the specialists' opinions and not to use medication due to fear of adverse effects, but underwent follow-up and observation. At 6 months after diagnosis, the patient was able to maintain normal activities in work and life, but still showed vertigo symptoms and frequent episodes of vertigo.

## 15.3 Case Review

Based on the patient's clinical presentation, the patient first needs to be considered for the presence of the following common vertigo disorders: (1) BPPV: Although the patient was not at BPPV-prone age, she was diagnosed with BPPV by the local hospital because she had recurrent episodes of positional vertigo for more than 2 years, transient vertigo episodes occurred mostly when getting up or lying down, and her symptom characteristics were very similar to those of persistent BPPV, and her positional test was positive, so the presence of other possible causes should be considered. (2) Vestibular migraine: Some patients with vestibular migraine may also present with positional vertigo symptoms as well as positional nystagmus, or even a positive Dix-Hallpike test. Therefore, it is important to interview the patient for headache symptoms, history of headache, history of motion sickness, and family history of related headache and motion sickness. This patient had no associated headache concomitant symptoms, so the diagnosis of vestibular migraine was not considered. (3) Meniere disease: A few patients with Meniere disease may also present with positional vertigo symptoms and positional nystagmus, but this patient had no cochlear symptoms such as deafness, tinnitus, or ear fullness, which does not support the diagnosis of Meniere disease. (4) Central positional vertigo and nystagmus: Because the patient had no other neurologic symptoms such as headache, convulsions, symptoms of impaired consciousness, diplopia, choking on water, or dysarthria, the clinician could not easily consider that the patient's positional vertigo and nystagmus manifestations were due to a central occupying lesion. However, the patient's multiple positional tests showed vertical down-beating nystagmus, and the features of her nystagmus presentation were suggestive of central positional nystagmus. A careful reading of the patient's brain MRI performed at the local hospital revealed the presence of a suspicious occupying lesion in the cerebellar vermis. Central paroxysmal positional vertigo is a group of paroxysmal positional vertigo of central origin. Common lesion sites include the dorsolateral part of the fourth ventricle, the dorsal cerebellar vermis, the cerebellar nodulus, and the lingual lobe. If the nystagmus induced by positional test does not correspond to a manifestation of excitation or inhibition of the corresponding semicircular canal, or if positional nystagmus occurs on multiple positional tests, but the responsible semicircular canal cannot be identified, brain MRI should be promptly performed to exclude central positional vertigo caused by a central lesion, especially an occupying lesion. In this patient, the presence of cerebellar vermis lesion was confirmed by further brain MRI and MRS, while the imaging features were consistent with low-grade glioma. After consultation with experts from several hospitals, the patient received a treatment opinion for observation and follow-up. At 6 months of follow-up, the patient was able to carry on with daily work and life, but her vertigo symptoms persisted and vertigo episodes were frequent. The patient should be closely followed up in the future and interventional treatment can be considered, if necessary.

## Bibliography

Bhattacharyya N, Gubbels SP, Schwartz SR, et al. Clinical practice guideline: benign paroxysmal positional vertigo (update). Otolaryngol Head Neck Surg. 2017;156(3):403–16.

Cho BH, Kim SH, Kim SS, et al. Central positional nystagmus associated with cerebellar tumors: clinical and topographical analysis. J Neurol Sci. 2017;373:147–51.

Macdonald NK, Kaski D, Saman Y, et al. Central positional nystagmus: a systematic literature review. Front Neurol. 2017;8:141.

Power L, Murray K, Drummond KJ, et al. Fourth ventricle ependymoma mimicking benign paroxysmal positional vertigo. Neurology. 2018;91(7):327–8.

Young AS, Lechner C, Bradshaw AP, et al. Capturing acute vertigo: a vestibular event monitor. Neurology. 2019;92(24):e2743–53.

# Meningioma of the Saddle Area Presenting as Recurrent Vertigo

16

Chunlin Zhang

## 16.1 Summary of Medical Records

Patient, female, 63 years old. Complaint: Recurrent episodes of vertigo for 20 years. Present history: 20 years ago, the patient had a sudden onset of vertigo without apparent cause, with a sensation of spinning vision, which lasted for a few minutes and then resolved without any specific treatment. Since then, vertigo attacks have occurred every few years with the same symptoms as before. The patient reported that she started to have tinnitus in her right ear 4–5 years before the onset of vertigo, but the tinnitus did not increase significantly after the onset of vertigo. And 16 years ago, she started to have hearing loss in her right ear, which was mild and was not treated, and no cranio-cerebral imaging had been done. The patient had recurrent episodes of vertigo once every 1–2 days, and the symptoms were worse than before, and the vertigo symptoms lasted for 3–5 min and resolved on their own. During the vertigo attack, the patient's deafness and tinnitus symptoms were not aggravated, and were not accompanied by headache, blackout, diplopia, numbness of limbs, weakness, convulsions, and disturbance of consciousness. The patient had no specific discomfort between episodes of vertigo and was able to perform daily tasks. She had been treated for Meniere disease at a local hospital, but her symptoms had not improved. The patient was admitted to the hospital on 21 November 2018 for further consultation. Physical examination: general examination and neurological examination did not show any abnormality. Otologic examination: bilateral external auditory canals and tympanic membranes were not abnormal, and spontaneous nystagmus was negative. However, 1 day after admission, the patient had a sudden onset of vertigo with unstable sitting and near-fall while turning her head to the left in a sitting position, and on examination at that time, III° rightward horizontal nystagmus lasting for about 1 min was observed. The following ancillary tests were performed after admission. Pure tone audiometry: mean hearing threshold of 77.5 dBHL in the right ear from 0.5 to 4 kHz, normal hearing threshold in the left ear. Tympanometry: both ear tympanograms showed normal type A curves. The acoustic reflex was not elicited by 0.5 and 1 kHz acoustic stimulation in the right ear, and the acoustic reflex was normal in the left ear. Auditory brainstem response (ABR): 30 dBHL threshold in the left ear and 70 dBHL threshold in the right ear, with fair differentiation of waves I-V in both ears. Cervical vestibular evoked myogenic potential (c-VEMP) detection: left $P_1$ latency 17.7 ms, $N_1$ latency 23.8 ms, $P_1$-$N_1$ amplitude 182.6 μV; right $P_1$ latency 14.3 ms, $N_1$ latency 22.2 ms, $P_1$-$N_1$ amplitude 73.0 μV, asymmetry ratio 42.9% on both sides. Nystagmogram: positive spontaneous

C. Zhang (✉)
Department of Neurology, Central Hospital of Liuzhou Railway, Liuzhou, China

© Scientific and Technical Documentation Press 2023

X. Shan, E. Wang (eds.), *Interpretation of Vertigo Cases*, Experts' Perspectives on Medical Advances, https://doi.org/10.1007/978-981-99-6995-1_16

nystagmus, presenting as rightward horizontal nystagmus, with slow phase velocity of 5.9°/s. The positional tests: the lying-down test showed rightward horizontal nystagmus with a slow phase velocity of 6.0°/s; both the left roll test and the left Dix-Hallpike test showed rightward horizontal nystagmus, with slow phase velocity of 5.9°/s or 6.0°/s, accompanied with vertical down-beating nystagmus, while both the right roll test and the right Dix-Hallpike test were negative. Velocity step test: showing the closed slow phase velocities of post-rotational nystagmus triggered by suddenly stopping after sustained rotation on both sides, with a CP value of 13.2%. Head-shaking test: showed rightward horizontality nystagmus with a slow phase velocity of 14°/s. Caloric test: mild paralysis of the right horizontal semicircular canal (CP = 25%), suggesting reduced function of the right horizontal semicircular canal. Visual dysmetria test: bilaterally undershoot. Visual smooth pursuit test: showing a type III curve. Optokinetic nystagmus test: no abnormality was seen. Gaze nystagmus: negative. Posturography: static posture map (eyes open and closed) with diffuse center of gravity, total track length of kinetic shaking was 63.7 and 71.7 cm, respectively; sponge pad (eyes open and closed) with diffuse distribution of center of gravity, total track length of kinetic shaking was 44.6 and 54.7 cm, respectively. Electrocochleography: SP/AP ratio was 0.58 in the right ear. Brain MRI scan: a mass was seen in the saddle area, with slightly long and more uniform $T_2$ signal, the bilateral cavernous sinuses were encircled by the mass lesion, the left anterior border of the pons was slightly compressed, the left trigeminal nerve was completely encircled, the roots of the left facial and auditory nerves were slightly compressed, the right facial and auditory nerves were normal, and the bilateral cochleae and semicircular canals were normal in shape (Fig. 16.1a). Brain MRI enhancement: showing an occupying lesion in the saddle area, with more obvious homogeneous enhancement, and the meningeal tail sign was visible around the lesion, considering the diagnosis of possible meningioma (Fig. 16.1b). The oncology radiotherapy department was consulted: meningioma was considered and surgery and postoperative local radiation therapy were recommended. However, the patient was unwilling to undergo surgery and radiotherapy, so she was discharged from the hospital and was closely followed up.

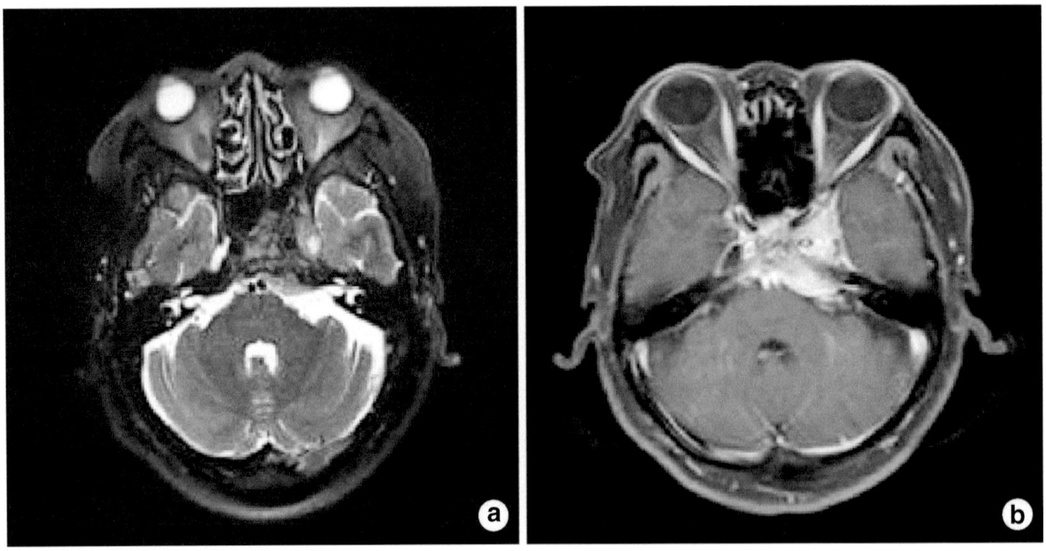


**Fig. 16.1** Brain MRI. (**a**) MRI plain scan; (**b**) MRI enhancement scan. An occupying lesion in the saddle area with homogeneous enhancement and a meningeal tail sign seen in the periphery of the lesion, suggesting a meningioma

## 16.2 Case Study

The saddle area is located at the base of the skull with complex anatomical structure. Above it are the optic cross, anterior cerebral artery, and anterior communicating artery; below it are the septum and pituitary gland; anteriorly is the optic nerve; posteriorly is the pituitary stalk and funnel; and on both sides are the internal carotid artery and posterior communicating artery. Brain tumors in the saddle area may have a variety of clinical presentations due to the complex neurovascular relationships surrounding the tumors. Meningiomas in the saddle area mostly have a slow onset and long course, and the symptoms at the beginning of the disease are mild and often neglected. With the passage of time, the tumor grows slowly and can encircle and compress the surrounding nerves, blood vessels, and other structures, and new clinical symptoms and signs appear one after another, and the degree of symptoms gradually increases. Most meningiomas in the saddle area have visual impairment, dizziness, and headache as the initial symptoms, and may have psychiatric symptoms, seizures, decreased sense of smell, and abnormal endocrine function symptoms such as amenorrhea, lactation, and decreased libido, while tinnitus, deafness, and vertigo symptoms are less common. In this case, the duration of the disease was more than 20 years, and the sequence of symptom evolution was as follows: tinnitus in the right ear, episodic vertigo, deafness in the right ear, and increased frequency of vertigo attacks with episodic unsteadiness in sitting, and falling down. The patient did not care about the tinnitus and deafness symptoms because they started insidiously and affected the patient's daily life to a lesser extent, but presented to the vertigo clinic with episodic vertigo as the main complaint. In the absence of brain MRI findings, the episodic nature of vertigo in this case seemed consistent with the diagnosis of probable vestibular paroxysmia, and the cause of deafness and tinnitus in the right ear was unknown. In contrast, the meningioma lesion in this case was showed by brain MRI, internal auditory meatus MRI, and brain MRA and its relationship with peripheral nerves could explain all symptoms and signs of the patient, so the diagnosis of meningioma in the saddle area was made by the principle of monism. The current treatment strategy for meningioma is mostly based on the guidelines published by the National Comprehensive Cancer Network (NCCN) and the European Association of Neuro-Oncology (EANO), and the treatment plan is established on the basis of the World Health Organization classification, with the degree of surgical resection measured by the Simpson classification criteria. Surgical resection is the treatment of choice for symptomatic meningiomas. The surgical principle is to preserve neurological function to the maximum extent and to remove the tumor tissue as completely as possible, while interventional or radiological treatment is given to residual tumor and recurrent tumor after surgery. In this case, the neurological deficit caused by meningioma continued to worsen, and the patient's general condition was good, so there were clear indications for surgery. In view of the special anatomical location of the tumor in the saddle area, the close relationship with the surrounding vessels and nerves and the size of the tumor, complete resection of the tumor could not be achieved by surgery, so the treatment plan of surgery combined with postoperative radiotherapy was recommended.

## 16.3 Case Review

The saddle area is located at the base of the skull, and the complex anatomic relation with surrounding tissues has a great influence on the growth pattern and clinical manifestations of meningioma in the saddle area. Therefore, meningioma in the saddle area can present a variety of clinical symptoms and signs, and the difficulty of surgical treatment increases due to the complex anatomical relationship between the tumor and surrounding blood vessels and nerves. As the tumor growth process advances, the more nerves and blood vessels are encircled and compressed by the meningioma in the saddle area, and the closer the relationship with the surrounding blood vessels and nerves is, the more difficult the surgery is, the more surgical complications there are, and the worse the surgical results are. Therefore, early detection of tumors is an important task for clinicians. However, the symptoms of meningioma in the saddle area are mild at the beginning of the disease and progress slowly, so the early symptoms are easily ignored by patients and doctors, and brain MRI is an indispensable diagnostic basis. Therefore, it is an essential task for clinicians to avoid underdiagnosis of early symptoms and to sort out the intrinsic connection of various symptoms during the long course of the disease, so as to derive the clinical decision of performing brain imaging. From the perspective of vertigo science, the importance of brain imaging for the diagnosis of patients with vertigo remains well illustrated in this case. The patient presented with episodic vertigo as the main complaint and had a history of vertigo for 20 years until the first brain MRI was performed at this visit, which revealed the meningioma in the saddle area was the cause of paroxysmal vertigo in this patient. This vertigo is a central vertigo, and also so-called malignant vertigo. The meningioma is of chronic course, and it is evident that the failure to perform brain imaging in the past could delay the detection of the tumor. Whether brain imaging should be used as a routine method and indication for screening for central dizziness or vertigo deserves further study.

## Bibliography

Karsy M, Sonnen J, Couldwell WT. Coincident pituitary adenoma and sellar meningioma. Acta Neurochir. 2015;157(2):231–3.

Wu M, Huo G, Yang G, et al. Clinical features and surgical treatment strategy of meningioma in the saddle area. J Chongqing Med Univ. 2015;40(1):88–91.

# 17 Vestibular Rehabilitation of Balance Dysfunction After Surgery of Vestibular Schwannoma

Huibing Wang and Jian Li

## 17.1 Summary of Medical Records

Patient, male, 39 years old. Complaint: Hearing loss and tinnitus in the left ear for more than 1 month. Present history: The patient began to have hearing loss in the left ear with persistent tinnitus 1 month ago. There was no significant hearing loss and tinnitus in the right ear. The patient had no symptoms of vertigo or dizziness and headache. Since the onset of the disease, there were no signs of blackout, impaired consciousness, numbness, and movement disorders in the limbs, or speech disorders. He was admitted to the hospital on April 11, 2017 for further diagnosis and treatment. Past history: no history of radiation exposure and no history of tumor. Admission examination: general condition was good, no positive signs were seen on general examination and neurological examination. Otologic examination: The external ear and tympanic membrane were normal bilaterally, and there was no erythema or pressure pain in the mastoid region. Pure tone audiometry: the left ear showed sensorineural deafness with pure tone air conduction hearing thresholds of 20 dBHL/0.5 kHz, 60 dBHL/1 kHz, 70 dBHL/2 kHz and 75 dBHL/4 kHz; the right ear hearing was basically normal. Tympanometry: bilateral tympanograms showed type A curves. Otoacoustic emissions: transient otoacoustic emissions and aberrant otoacoustic emissions were elicited in the right ear, while transient otoacoustic emissions and aberrant otoacoustic emissions were not elicited in the left ear. Auditory brainstem response (ABR): 80 dBHL response threshold in the left ear, slight delay in waves III and V; 30 dBHL response threshold in the right ear, normal latency in waves I–V. Vestibular function examination: negative for spontaneous nystagmus. Caloric test: showing the reduced function of the left horizontal semicircular canal, with mild canal paralysis (CP = 50%). CT of the temporal bone: no abnormalities were seen. MRI and enhanced MRI of the internal auditory meatus: an occupying lesion showed in the left internal auditory meatus, approximately 13 mm × 19 mm in size, which was considered to be a vestibular schwannoma (acoustic neuroma), with cystic changes within the tumor (Fig. 17.1). Clinical diagnosis: left-sided vestibular schwannoma. The patient under general anesthesia underwent the resection of the vestibular schwannoma via a retrosigmoid approach. Postoperative pathology: left vestibular schwannoma. Postoperatively, the patient had complete hearing loss in the left ear with dizziness and unsteadiness in walking, but no sense of visual rotation. The patient was followed up by telephone for 1 year after surgery, except for deafness in the left ear, the symptoms of unsteadi-

H. Wang · J. Li (✉)
Institute of Vertigo, Third Medical Center, PLA General Hospital, Beijing, China

© Scientific and Technical Documentation Press 2023

X. Shan, E. Wang (eds.), *Interpretation of Vertigo Cases*, Experts' Perspectives on Medical Advances, https://doi.org/10.1007/978-981-99-6995-1_17

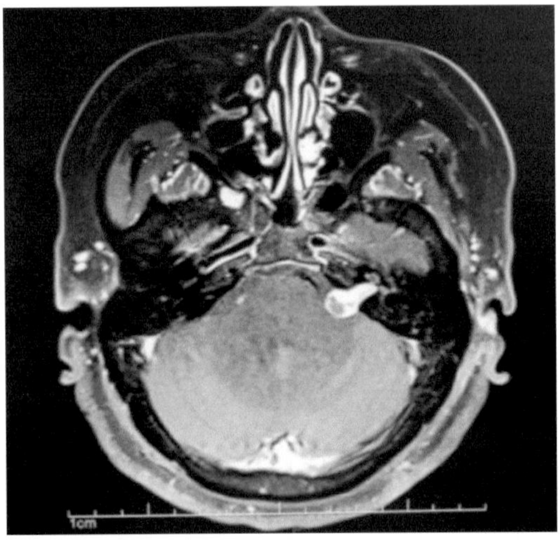


**Fig. 17.1** Brain MRI. Axial $T_1$ image shows a left-sided vestibular schwannoma measuring approximately 13 mm × 19 mm, involving the internal auditory meatus and cerebellopontine angle, with cystic changes within the tumor

ness were significantly improved, and no tumor recurrence was seen on head CT.

## 17.2 Case Study

This patient had left tinnitus with hearing loss for 1 month, and his hearing loss was unilateral and progressive with tinnitus symptoms. His audiological examination showed high frequency hearing loss in the left ear, and auditory brainstem-evoked potential testing showed an increased response threshold in the left ear (80 dBHL) with slightly delayed waves III and V. Vestibular function examination showed reduced function of the left horizontal semicircular canal, but preoperatively, the patient did not have significant symptoms of vertigo or dizziness and imbalance. There were no signs of facial nerve, trigeminal nerve, or other cranial nerve damage, except for the auditory nerve damage. Enhanced MRI showed an occupying lesion in the internal auditory meatus and the cerebellopontine angle. Both imaging and clinical diagnoses were (left) vestibular schwannoma. Examination suggested that the vestibular schwannoma involved the cochlear nerve and vestibular nerve. Progressive hearing loss is the most common clinical manifestation of acoustic neuroma (vestibular schwannoma), accounting for about 95% of cases and it may be caused by compression of the cochlear nerve or involvement of the blood supply to the cochlea, mainly manifesting as unilateral or asymmetric progressive hearing loss, mostly involving firstly the high frequencies. And the hearing loss due to vestibular schwannoma can also manifest as sudden hearing loss, which can be caused by spasm or obstruction of the internal auditory artery due to tumor compression. Tinnitus accounts for about 70% of cases and is predominantly a high-frequency tone. Vertigo can be recurrent, mostly as non-rotational vertigo, but predominantly with the symptoms of instability and imbalance in walking, mostly appearing in the early growth stages of vestibular schwannoma, as a result of vestibular nerve or labyrinthine blood supply involvement, and the symptoms can gradually decrease or disappear with vestibular function compensation. According to the size of the tumor, those with a diameter of <2.5 cm are considered as small vestibular schwannoma. In this case, surgery was chosen because the vestibular schwannoma had involved and compressed the cerebellopontine angle and was accompanied by cystic change in nature. After surgery, the patient showed symptoms of vestibular dysfunction such as dizziness and unstable walking, which were gradually reduced by vestibular rehabilitation exercises, and the symptoms of postural instability were significantly improved 1 year after surgery.

## 17.3 Case Review

Acoustic neuroma, also called vestibular schwannoma because this tumor mostly originates from the vestibular nerve, is a benign tumor and accounts for 80–90% of tumors in the pontocerebellar angle. The tumor can originate from any branch of the auditory-vestibular nerve. With the growth of the tumor, it gradually compresses the surrounding important structures and nerves, including the auditory-vestibular nerve, facial nerve, trigeminal nerve, abducens nerve, posterior group of cranial nerves, cerebellum, brain stem, etc., thus producing the corresponding symptoms. In the early stage, tinnitus, sensorineural hearing loss and unsteady walking may occur due to the involvement of the auditory-vestibular nerve, while the symptoms of other cranial nerve injury such as peripheral facial palsy may appear in the middle and late stages. These symptoms are non-specific and can be easily overlooked or misdiagnosed. In this case, the patient presented with tinnitus in the left ear with hearing loss for more than 1 month, and audiological examination showed sensorineural deafness in his left ear with predominantly high-frequency hearing loss, which could easily be diagnosed as neurogenic deafness and tinnitus. Early vestibular schwannoma often does not show significant enlargement of the internal auditory meatus due to the small size of the tumor, and CT may not show any abnormality. In contrast, ABR and MRI have a high rate of diagnosis of small vestibular schwannoma. In the early stages of auditory nerve pathogenesis, ABR can be used as a screening test for its diagnosis and may show a prolonged V-wave latency. In addition, tinnitus symptoms often go unnoticed because they do not seriously affect the patient's work and life. Unilateral hearing loss without tinnitus, or unilateral tinnitus with mild hearing loss, especially if it is not accompanied by vertigo symptoms, is easily overlooked. Some patients only discover unilateral hearing loss when they are on the phone. Therefore, there should be sufficient awareness of the early manifestations of vestibular schwannoma to enable timely diagnosis and treatment of the tumor. Those with unilateral tinnitus and unilateral hearing loss, especially those with predominant hearing loss in the middle and high frequencies, should be highly alert to the possibility of vestibular schwannoma.

## Bibliography

Mackeith SA, Kerr RS, Milford CA. Trends in acoustic neuroma management: a 20-year review of the oxford skull base clinic. J Neurol Surg B Skull Base. 2013;74(4):194–200.

McClelland S 3rd, Kim E, Murphy JD, et al. Operative mortality rates of acoustic neuroma surgery: a National Cancer Database analysis. Otol Neurotol. 2017;38(5):751–3.

Monfared A, Corrales CE, Theodosopoulos PV, et al. Facial nerve outcome and tumor control rate as a function of degree of resection in treatment of large acoustic neuromas: preliminary report of the acoustic neuroma subtotal resection study (ANSRS). Neurosurgery. 2016;79(2):194–203.

Tolisano AM, Burgos RM, Lustik MB, et al. Asymmetric hearing loss prompting MRI referral in a military population: redefining audiometric criteria. Otolaryngol Head Neck Surg. 2018;158(4):695–701.

# 18 Cavernous Hemangioma of the Pontine Arm with Positional Vertigo as the First Symptom

Juanli Xing

## 18.1 Summary of Medical Records

Patient, female, 65 years old. Complaint: Vertigo for 6 months, unstable walking with vomiting for half a month. Present history: 6 months ago, the patient experienced dizziness when she lowered or raised her head, or changed her body position, occasionally with vision rotate, and felt hearing loss in her left ear, but no tinnitus or ear fullness. She was diagnosed with cervical spondylosis and cerebral blood supply deficiency at the local hospital and given symptomatic treatment, which was not effective. The patient came to our hospital on January 11, 2016. Past history: no history of hypertension, diabetes mellitus, no history of smoking or alcoholism. Physical examination: no significant abnormality on general physical examination. No significant abnormalities were seen on brain CT examination prior to consultation. Pure tone audiometry: mild sensorineural deafness in both ears, with basically symmetry on both sides at mean hearing thresholds around 40 dBHL. Auditory brainstem response (ABR): tone burst stimulation of 80 dBHL in the right ear elicited wave I, wave III, and wave V with good waveform differentiation and no significant prolongation of latency, but tone burst stimulation of 100 dBHL in the left ear elicited wave I, wave III, or wave V. Vestibular function examination: saccade test, smooth pursuit test and optokinetic test all showed normal; caloric test results were not significantly abnormal, and visual fixation suppression test was positive. Vestibular autorotation test (VAT): increased horizontal gain, suggesting central vestibular injury; bilateral Dix-Hallpike tests induced vertical down-beating nystagmus without torsional nystagmus component; supine roll test was negative. MRI of the internal auditory meatus (Fig. 18.1): a heterogeneous $T_1$ WI and $T_2$ WI mixed high signal shadow was seen at the left pontine arm, a $T_2$ WI low signal shadow was seen at the edge of the lesion, and a DWI image showed a slightly high signal shadow surrounded by a low signal shadow at the edge of the lesion. MRI diagnosis: cavernous hemangioma of the left pontine arm. The patient was then transferred to our radiotherapy center for further treatment. The patient underwent craniotomy and removal of tumor under general anesthesia on January 15, 2016. Postoperative pathology: cavernous hemangioma. One month later the patient was discharged in stable condition and did not complain of any special discomfort. At follow-up 3 months after discharge, the patient's previous symptoms disappeared, no more vertigo episodes when changing body position or head position, and a repeat VAT showed normal vestibular function. The patient's condition is well.

J. Xing (✉)
Department of Otolaryngology, Head and Neck Surgery, First Affiliated Hospital, School of Medicine, Xi'an Jiaotong University, Xi'an, China

© Scientific and Technical Documentation Press 2023
X. Shan, E. Wang (eds.), *Interpretation of Vertigo Cases*, Experts' Perspectives on Medical Advances, https://doi.org/10.1007/978-981-99-6995-1_18

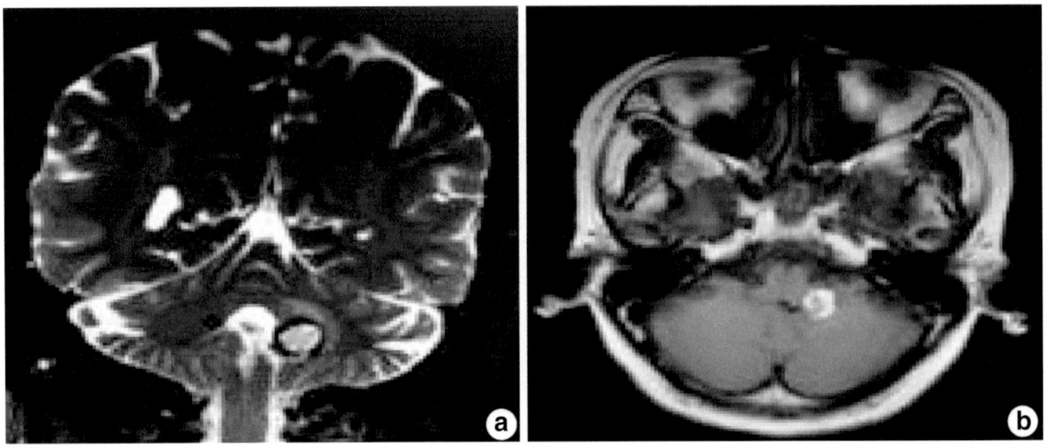


**Fig. 18.1** MRI of the internal auditory meatus and brain. Cavernous hemangioma in the left pontine arm. (**a**) coronal view; (**b**) horizontal view

## 18.2 Case Study

The patient was an elderly female who started to have positional vertigo 6 months ago when she lowered or raised her head and changed her body position. The audiological examination showed that the pure tone hearing threshold was mildly increased in both ears, but the hearing was basically symmetrical on both sides. ABR showed no significant abnormality in the right ear, while it did not show the wave I, wave III, or wave V in the left ear. The disappearance of wave V suggested a possible auditory neuroma or brainstem tumor lesion. The Dix-Hallpike test induced vertical downbeat nystagmus bilaterally without a torsional nystagmus component. Therefore, it was suspected that the patient's positional vertigo or nystagmus might be due to a central disorder, and an MRI of the internal auditory meatus was performed and the diagnosis of cavernous hemangioma in the left pontine arm was made. The patient was treated promptly and had a good outcome.

## 18.3 Case Review

Spongiform hemangiomas are not true tumors and are vascular malformations of the brain, most of which are congenital anomalies. Spongiform hemangiomas can occur anywhere in the brain and can cause epilepsy, hemorrhage, and neurological deficits, with recurrent intracranial hemorrhage being the main cause of symptoms from the disease. Brainstem cavernous hemangiomas account for approximately 20% of intracranial cavernous hemangiomas and occur mostly in the pons. The pontine arm forms the midfoot of the cerebellum, which is the connection between the cerebellum and the pons. Because the nuclei of the V–VIII pairs of cranial nerves reside in the pons, the lesions in pontine arm can lead to pontine arm syndrome, typically presenting with the symptoms of damage to the trigeminal nerve, sphenoid nerve, facial nerve, and vestibulocochlear nerve on the side of the lesion. Damage to the vestibulocochlear nerve can lead to deafness and balance dysfunction. The high prevalence of vertigo and the complex etiology and pathogenesis of vertiginous disorders sometimes make diagnosis and differential diagnosis difficult, and some central vertigo caused by intracranial occupational lesions are easily misdiagnosed.

## Bibliography

Brandt T, Dieterich M. The dizzy patient: don't forget disorders of the central vestibular system. Nat Neurol Rev. 2017;13(6):352–62.

Choi JY, Kim JH, Kim HJ, et al. Central paroxysmal positional nystagmus: characteristics and possible mechanisms. Neurology. 2015;84(22):2238–46.
Donnelly JP, Chancellor AM, El-Dieb A. Central cause of positioning vertigo. Pract Neurol. 2018;18(6):492–3.
Macdonald NK, Kaski D, Saman Y, et al. Central positional nystagmus: a systematic literature review. Front Neurol. 2017;8:141.

# 19 Cerebellar Aneurysm with Acute Cerebellar Infarction Causing Episodic Vertigo

Qinghua Zhang

## 19.1 Summary of Medical Records

Patient, male, 31 years old. Complaint: episodes of vertigo for 5 days. Present history: The patient had a sudden onset of vertigo with no obvious cause 5 days ago, with rotating vision, accompanied by nausea, vomiting, and unstable walking. Since the onset, the patient had no aural symptoms such as tinnitus, ear fullness, hearing loss, or neurological manifestations such as headache, amaurosis, diplopia, facial palsy, speech dysfluency, twitching of limbs, or disturbance of consciousness. Past history: previously healthy, no history of hypertension, hyperlipidemia, heart disease, etc. Admission examination: no abnormalities were found on general examination. Bilateral tendon reflexes were normal, pathological reflexes were not elicited, finger-nose test and heel-knee-tibial test were stable and accurate. Otologic examination: external auditory canal and tympanic membrane were normal. Pure tone audiometry: hearing was normal in both ears. Tympanometry: showed normal type A tympanic curves in both ears; the stapedial muscle acoustic reflexes in both ears could be elicited normally. Auditory brainstem response (ABR): binaural thresholds of 30 dBHL, each wave could be elicited with good repeatability, and the I-V wave interval was normal. Vestibular function examination: negative for spontaneous nystagmus. Visual oculomotor test: normal. Caloric test: normal bilateral horizontal semicircular canal function. VEMP: reduced amplitude in the left ear, interaural asymmetry ratio 21.5%. Positional tests: bilateral Dix-Hallpike tests were negative, but supine roll test was positive, showing apogeotropic direction-changed positional nystagmus, indicating a diagnosis of the cupulolithiasis of the left horizontal semicircular canal. However, the patient's symptoms were still present after repositioning treatment. Electrocardiogram and cardiac ultrasound examination showed no significant abnormal findings. Brain MRI: showed acute infarction of the cerebellar vermis and left cerebellar hemisphere. The neurology consultation diagnosed as acute cerebellar infarction, and the patient was treated with medications, including edaravone, sodium ozagrelate, prostaglandin injection, and butalbital peptide. Further head and neck CTA examination suggested a left cerebellar aneurysm (Fig. 19.1). Thus, the patient was referred to neurovascular surgery for further review and treatment. Whole-brain angiography with local anesthesia revealed an aneurysm in the fourth segment of the left posterior inferior cerebellar artery, and the next day intracranial aneurysm embolization was

Q. Zhang (✉)
Institute of Vertigo, Third Medical Center, PLA General Hospital, Beijing, China

© Scientific and Technical Documentation Press 2023
X. Shan, E. Wang (eds.), *Interpretation of Vertigo Cases*, Experts' Perspectives on Medical Advances, https://doi.org/10.1007/978-981-99-6995-1_19

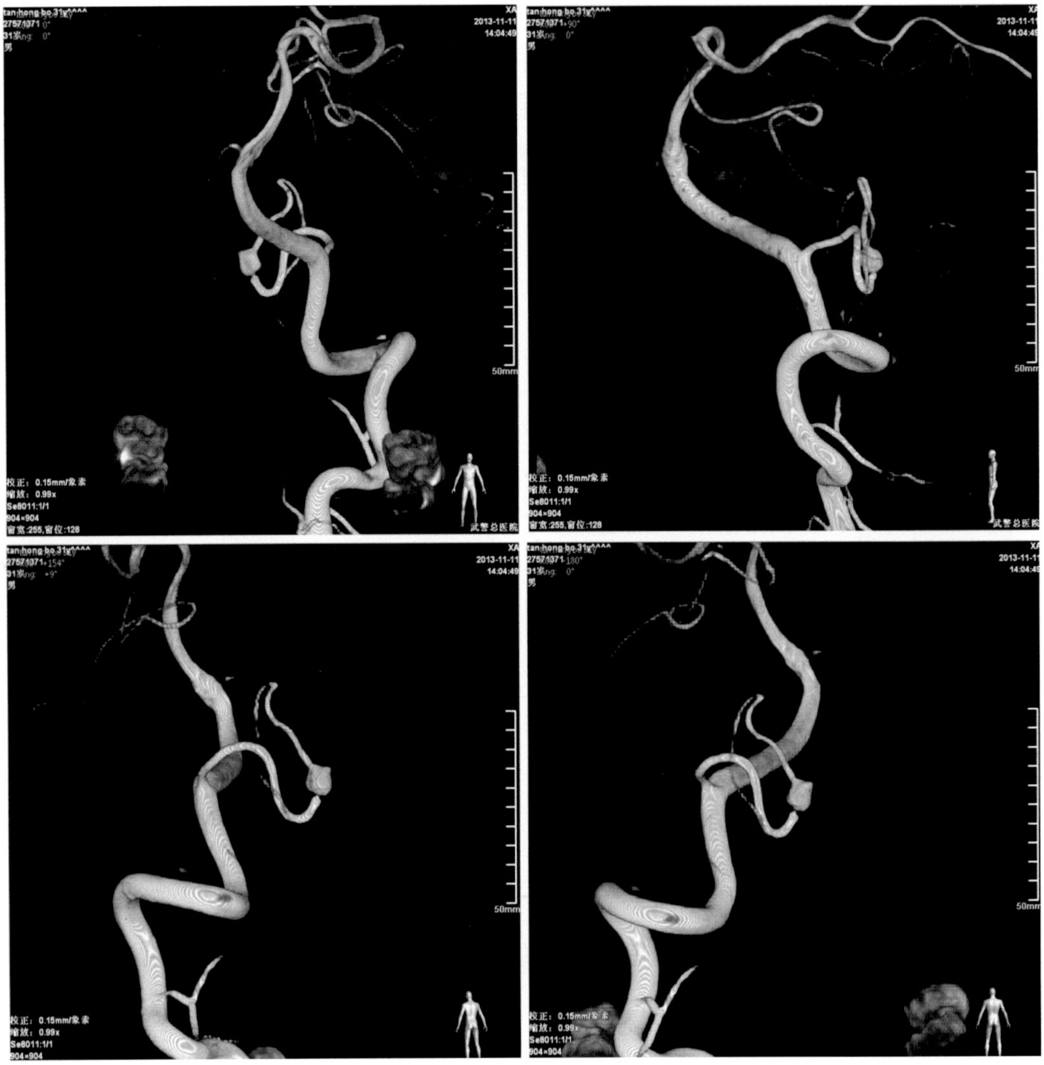


**Fig. 19.1** Cerebral angiography. A spindle-shaped dilatation and an aneurysm were showed in the fourth segment of the left posterior inferior cerebellar artery

performed under general anesthesia and the aneurysm-carrying artery of the posterior inferior cerebellar artery was occluded with a spring coil (Fig. 19.2). The patient recovered well after the operation and he is currently in good condition.

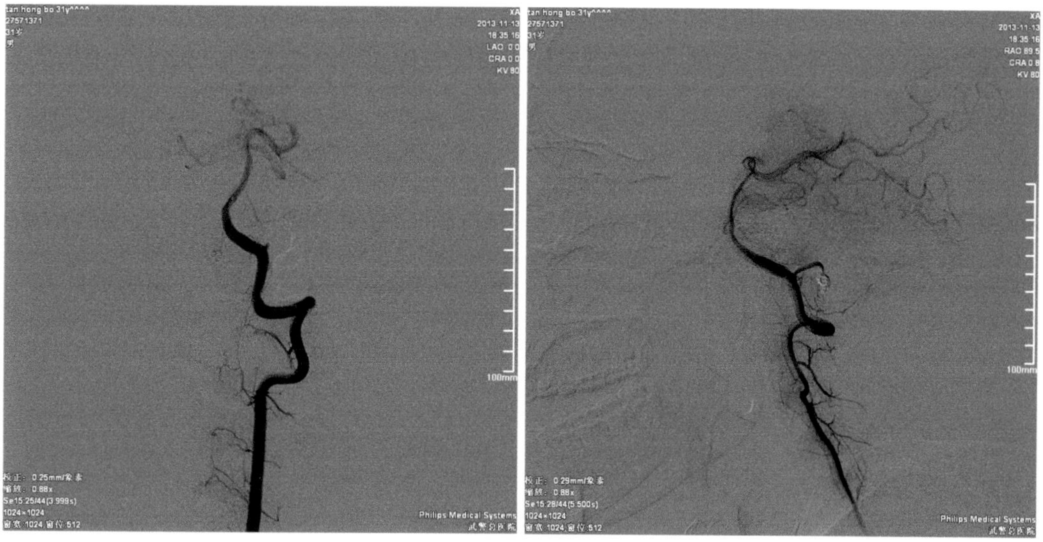

**Fig. 19.2** Cerebral angiography and aneurysm embolization. The aneurysm-carrying artery of the left posterior inferior cerebellar artery was occluded with a spring coil

## 19.2 Case Study

The patient was a young male who presented with episodes of vertigo for 5 days with no apparent cause, accompanied by symptoms of nausea, vomiting, and unsteadiness in walking. The patient did not have the symptoms of hearing loss, tinnitus, ear fullness, and headache since the onset of the disease. He was in good health and had no risk factors for cardiovascular or cerebrovascular diseases. The patient presented with an acute vertigo attack, and it was firstly considered whether his vertigo attack was due to common vertigo disorders such as Meniere disease, vestibular migraine, vestibular neuritis, and benign paroxysmal positional vertigo (BPPV), and differential diagnoses are required. Meniere disease presents with recurrent episodes of vertigo with deafness, tinnitus, and ear fullness. The duration of vertigo episodes usually does not exceed 12 h, and hearing tests usually show hearing loss. The characteristics of clinical manifestations in this patient were inconsistent with Meniere disease. The main clinical symptom of vestibular migraine is recurrent episodes of vertigo with migraine manifestations, and this patient did not have the clinical manifestations of vestibular migraine either. Vestibular neuritis is mostly due to viral infection and may have prodromal manifestations of upper respiratory tract infection. Its clinical features are severe vertigo attacks with marked nausea and vomiting, with more severe symptoms of balance disturbance, and patient is often afraid to move around for fear of triggering a vertigo attack, and symptoms may gradually decrease over several days. However, the patient's spontaneous nystagmus was negative, and the caloric test showed normal bilateral vestibular functions, so it was not consistent with vestibular neuritis. BPPV is characterized by transient episodes of vertigo induced by specific head position changes and recurrent episodes of vertigo, with each episode usually lasting no more than 1 min or slightly longer than 1 min, while the patient's vertigo episodes were not closely related to head position changes and were persistent. The diagnosis of BPPV was not supported by the persistent nature of the vertigo episodes. Apogeotropic horizontal direction-changed positional nystagmus is not unique to BPPV and can be seen in some central lesions. Therefore, the patient was diagnosed with acute cerebellar infarction and treated promptly after imaging to determine whether the nystagmus was due to a central lesion. Further head and neck CTA and cerebral angiography revealed an aneurysm in the left posterior inferior cerebellar artery, which was treated with embolization of the posterior inferior cerebellar artery under general anesthesia to eliminate the potential risk for recurrent cerebellar infarction. The patient recovered well after the operation.

## 19.3 Case Review

Cerebellar infarction is a common central disease, a common type of posterior circulation infarction, in which hypertension, atherosclerosis, diabetes mellitus, heart disease, atrial fibrillation, dyslipidemia, and smoking are common causative factors, and a few cases are associated with aneurysms and thrombosis. Aneurysms occurring in the superior cerebellar artery, anterior inferior cerebellar artery, distal to the posterior inferior cerebellar artery and artery away from the ring of Willis and vertebrobasilar trunk are generally referred to as distal aneurysms. Digital subtraction angiography (DSA) is the gold standard for the diagnosis of aneurysms and can clearly show the location, size, and morphology of the aneurysm, accurately measure the width of the aneurysm neck, determine the type of aneurysm and the spatial anatomical relationship between the aneurysm and the aneurysm-carrying artery and its branches, provide an important basis for further treatment selection, and effectively offer early interventional treatment to avoid the recurrence of posterior circulation infarction.

## Bibliography

Blasberg TF, Wolf L, Henke C, et al. Isolated transient vertigo: posterior circulation ischemia or benign origin. BMC Neurol. 2017;17(1):111.

Chen YS, Sun C, Shi LA, et al. A report of 11 cases of posterior circulation infarction starting with isolated vertigo. J Clin Otolaryngol Head Neck Surg. 2018;32(7):547–50.

Choi JY, Lee SH, Kim JS. Central vertigo. Curr Opin Neurol. 2018;31(1):81–9.

Doijiri R, Uno H, Miyashita K, et al. How commonly is stroke found in patients with isolated vertigo or dizziness attack. J Stroke Cerebrovasc Dis. 2016;25(10):2549–52.

Wu C, Sun Z, Wang F, et al. Surgical treatment of intracranial distal aneurysms. Chin J Med. 2014;94(9):698–700.

# 20 Central Positional Vertigo Due to Cerebellar Infarction

Haijin Yi

## 20.1 Summary of Medical Records

Patient, male, 73 years old. Complaint: recurrent episodes of vertigo for 3 days. Present history: Three days ago, the patient had an episode of vertigo with nausea and vomiting during the change of body position, and had been seen at other hospital, considered as having benign paroxysmal positional vertigo (BPPV) and treated with canalith repositioning maneuvers and oral betahistine mesylate medication. The patient was brought to our emergency department by emergency vehicle due to sudden onset of severe vertigo with nausea, vomiting, and unsteadiness in standing and fainting when he woke up to use the toilet at night. The patient had no significant hearing loss or tinnitus since the onset, and had no significant headache or other neurological symptoms. Past history: The patient had a history of hypertension and diabetes mellitus, no history of coronary heart disease, trauma, and ear-related diseases. Emergency examination: both external auditory canals and tympanic membranes were normal. Positional test: Dix-Hallpike test was negative, but supine roll test was positive, showing apogeotropic horizontal nystagmus when patient turned his head to the left or right, with more pronounced nystagmus on rightward roll and lasting more than 1 min. The patient was treated with Barbecue repositioning maneuver according to cupulolithiasis of the horizontal semicircular canal BPPV, but the patient did not feel any significant improvement in the symptoms of positional vertigo and the nystagmus did not diminish significantly after repositioning treatments, so further audiological and vestibular function examinations were performed. Pure-tone audiometry: the hearing loss was characterized by age-related hearing loss, with mild high-frequency hearing loss and basically symmetry in both ears. Tympanometry: both tympanograms were type A curves. Nystagmographic examination: vertical up-beating spontaneous nystagmus, about 3°/s, could be recorded (Fig. 20.1); saccade function was basically normal; visual smooth pursuit test showed grade II–III curve; optokinetic nystagmus was basically normal. Caloric test: bilateral horizontal semicircular canal functions were normal. No significant abnormalities were seen on the video head impulse test. The patient was suspected to have central positional vertigo or nystagmus, so MRI was performed, suggesting a right cerebellar infarct foci, and he was referred to the neurology department for further treatments.

H. Yi (✉)
Department of Otolaryngology, Head and Neck Surgery, Beijing Tsinghua Changgung Hospital, Tsinghua University, Beijing, China

© Scientific and Technical Documentation Press 2023

X. Shan, E. Wang (eds.), *Interpretation of Vertigo Cases*, Experts' Perspectives on Medical Advances, https://doi.org/10.1007/978-981-99-6995-1_20

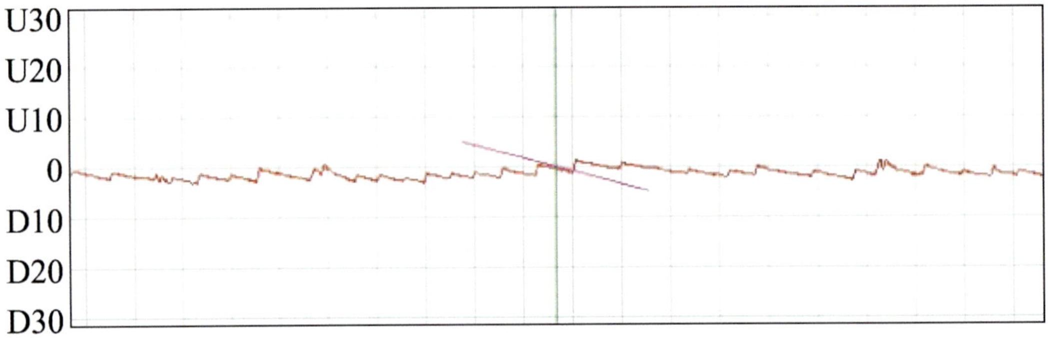


**Fig. 20.1** Nystagmography. Positive spontaneous nystagmus with vertical up-beating nystagmus

## 20.2 Case Study

The patient was an elderly male who presented with symptoms of postural change-related vertigo with nausea and vomiting, with no significant hearing loss or tinnitus symptoms, no significant headache or other neurological symptoms since the onset. He had been treated successively at two other hospitals for BPPV, but no significant effect was received. The patient was brought to our emergency department by ambulance because of sudden onset of severe vertigo with nausea, vomiting, unsteadiness, and fainting when waking up at night to use the toilet. The patient had a previous history of hypertension, diabetes, and other risk factors for cerebrovascular disease. The nystagmus was similar to the nystagmus of cupulolithiasis of the horizontal semicircular canal BPPV, and was treated with barbecue repositioning maneuver. However, after treatment, the patient did not feel any significant improvement in the symptoms of positional vertigo and the nystagmus did not diminish significantly. On further nystagmographic examination, the patient showed vertical up-beating spontaneous nystagmus. Visual smooth pursuit test findings showed grade II-III curve, while the caloric test indicated normal bilateral horizontal semicircular canal functions, and also the video head impulse test did not show any significant abnormality. Thus it was considered that the positional vertigo and nystagmus in this patient may be of central origin, which was confirmed with a following brain MRI, indicating cerebellar infarction. The patient's positional vertigo and nystagmus completely disappeared at 1 week after pharmacal treatments for cerebellar infarction. This case was diagnosed and treated in a timely manner and received a good treatment result.

## 20.3 Case Review

Positional vertigo or nystagmus can be caused by both peripheral and central lesions, with peripheral positional vertigo or nystagmus predominating and central positional vertigo or nystagmus being relatively uncommon. Peripheral positional vertigo or nystagmus is most commonly associated with BPPV, which is the most common form of peripheral vertigo and can account for 20% to 40% of vertigo cases. If you are familiar with the clinical features of BPPV, its diagnosis is not difficult and the disease can be treated well by the repositioning maneuver. Common diseases that cause central positional vertigo or nystagmus include: (1) posterior circulation cerebrovascular diseases, such as infarction of the anterior inferior cerebellar artery; (2) brain tumors, such as cerebellar tumors; (3) multiple sclerosis; and (4) familial ataxia. Although the incidence of central positional vertigo or nystagmus is low, it should be widely noted by clinicians because it is easily misdiagnosed as BPPV and can have serious consequences, therefore the two diseases need to be

**Table 20.1** Key points for differentiation between central positional vertigo and BPPV

| Characteristics of nystagmus and symptoms | BPPV | Central positional vertigo |
|---|---|---|
| Latency of nystagmus | 0 to several seconds | Often no latency |
| Duration of nystagmus | <1 min (canalolithiasis)<br>>1 min (cupulolithiasis) | Often persistent |
| Direction of nystagmus | Vertical rotational nystagmus on the Dix-Hallpike test (posterior or superior semicircular canal BPPV); or horizontal nystagmus on the roll test (horizontal semicircular canal BPPV) | Vertical nystagmus alone or in combination with head position change induced nystagmus |
| Fatigability of nystagmus | Mostly with fatigability | Rare with fatigability |
| Symptoms of vertigo | Vertigo mostly stops when nystagmus disappears | Vertigo and nystagmus do not always start and stop simultaneously |

differentiated (Table 20.1). Although most patients with central positional vertigo or nystagmus have neurological symptoms, there are still a few patients with isolated vertigo, i.e., vertigo symptoms without neurological symptoms, whose vertigo or nystagmus manifestations are very similar to those of BPPV. This requires the clinician to take a detailed history and physical examination, perform the necessary audiological, vestibular, and imaging examinations and assessments, and to be alert to the possibility of central positional vertigo or nystagmus when rare or atypical positional nystagmus is encountered, so that the patient can be diagnosed and treated in a timely and correct manner.

## Bibliography

Blasberg TF, Wolf L, Henke C, et al. Isolated transient vertigo: posterior circulation ischemia or benign origin? BMC Neurol. 2017;17(1):111.

Chen YS, Sun C, Shi LA, et al. A report of 11 cases of posterior circulation infarction starting with isolated vertigo. J Clin Otolaryngol Head Neck Surg. 2018;32(7):547–50.

Choi JY, Lee SH, Kim JS. Central vertigo. Curr Opin Neurol. 2018;31(1):81–9.

Doijiri R, Uno H, Miyashita K, et al. How commonly is stroke found in patients with isolated vertigo or dizziness attack. J Stroke Cerebrovasc Dis. 2016;25(10):2549–52.

Donnelly JP, Chancellor AM, El-Dieb A. Central cause of positioning vertigo. Pract Neurol. 2018;18(6):492–3.

# 21 Basilar Artery Aneurysm with Pontine Arm Infarction Presenting as Acute Cochleo-Vestibular Syndrome

Qinghua Zhang

## 21.1 Summary of Medical Records

Patient, male, 54 years old. Complaint: sudden onset of vertigo, hearing loss, and tinnitus for 10 h. Present history: The patient had a sudden onset of vertigo at 3:00 a.m. with rotating vision, accompanied by significant hearing loss and tinnitus in the right ear, and symptoms of nausea and vomiting, but no manifestations of impaired consciousness, blackout, diplopia, dysarthria, or speech dysfluency. The patient was admitted to the hospital with a diagnosis of sudden deafness with vertigo and was treated with medication to improve his cerebral circulation and vertigo symptom after emergency brain CT was performed to exclude cerebral hemorrhage because the patient had a history of hypertension, but the vertigo and ear symptoms did not improve significantly. Examinations: poor mental state, no abnormalities in general system examination, bilateral frontal lines and nasolabial folds were symmetrical, no down-turning of the corners of the mouth, left side facial sensation was normal, but with hypoesthesia of right face. The muscle strength and tone of the limbs were normal, and the ataxia test was normal. Cervical resistance was negative, bilateral Babinski's signs were negative. Neuro-otological examination: negative spontaneous nystagmus, no abnormality of bilateral external auditory canals and tympanic membranes. Pure tone audiometry: complete deafness in the right ear and normal hearing in the left ear. Tympanometry: both tympanograms showed normal type-A curves. Stapedial muscle acoustic reflex: not elicited in the right ear by ipsilateral stimuli, but elicited by contralateral stimuli at each frequency; elicited in the left ear by ipsilateral stimuli at each frequency, but not elicited by contralateral stimulation. Initial diagnosis: sudden deafness with vertigo. After admission, further cranial CT examination showed nodal shadow in the basilar artery area, and basilar artery aneurysm was considered. Brain MRI showed a basilar artery entrapment aneurysm with slightly high signal on DWI of the right pontine arm (Fig. 21.1). A digital subtraction whole brain angiography (DSA) showed multiple intracranial aneurysms, basilar artery entrapment aneurysm, and right anterior inferior cerebellar artery (AICA) occlusion. High-resolution MRI imaging of the basilar artery showed a basilar artery entrapment aneurysm with uneven thickness of the true lumen wall, demonstrating infarction in the pontine and right pontine arm (Fig. 21.2). The patient was diagnosed with a basilar artery entrapment aneurysm with acute pontine arm infarction. He was treated with stenting of the basilar artery entrapment aneurysm and postoperative symptomatic supportive therapy, including antiplatelet aggregation, fluid

Q. Zhang (✉)
Institute of Vertigo, Third Medical Center, PLA General Hospital, Beijing, China

© Scientific and Technical Documentation Press 2023
X. Shan, E. Wang (eds.), *Interpretation of Vertigo Cases*, Experts' Perspectives on Medical Advances, https://doi.org/10.1007/978-981-99-6995-1_21

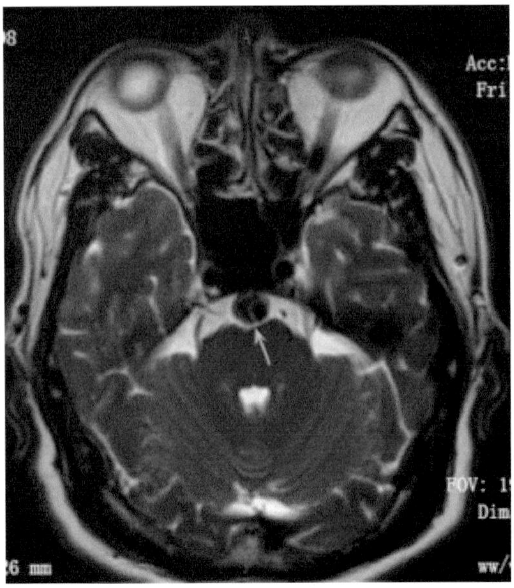


**Fig. 21.1** Brain MRI. The arrow shows a round-like signal shadow in the basilar artery area, with visible entrapment and a larger pseudo-lumen than the true lumen, and a circular short $T_1$ slightly long $T_2$ signal shadow in the wall of the true lumen, and an iso-$T_1$ short $T_2$ signal shadow in the pseudo-lumen, with compression of the adjacent pontine

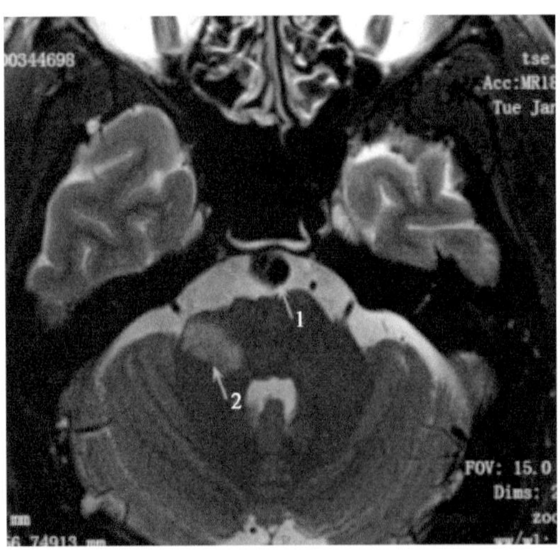


**Fig. 21.2** High-resolution MRI of brain blood vessels. Arrow 1 shows thickening of the lumen of the basilar artery with visible entrapment and a large pseudo-lumen with an arcuate inhomogeneous high-low signal; arrow 2 shows speckled, patchy long $T_1$ long $T_2$ signal in the pontine and right pontine arm

replacement, neurotrophy, and anti-vasospasm drugs. After treatment, the patient was discharged from the hospital with stable condition and gradual relief of vertigo symptoms. The patient was advised to adopt low-salt and low-fat diet, take regular medication, control blood pressure, avoid exertion and emotional excitement, and review regularly after discharge. The DSA review 5 months after stenting of the basilar artery coarctation aneurysm showed that the treatment result was satisfactory, and the patient did not have any recurrence of vertigo, but the hearing in the right ear did not improve significantly.

## 21.2 Case Study

The patient was a middle-aged male who presented to the emergency room with acute sudden vertigo, hearing loss and tinnitus in the right ear, without neurological localization signs. After excluding cerebral hemorrhage by emergency brain CT because of patient's hypertension history, he was treated with medications to improve cerebral circulation and vertigo symptoms, but the vertigo and ear symptoms did not improve significantly. Then the patient was considered as having sudden deafness with vertigo because his audiological examination findings were also consistent with sensorineural hearing loss on the one side and was admitted to the hospital for further diagnosis and treatment. The following brain MRI showed a basilar artery coarctation aneurysm with a slightly high DWI signal in the right pontine arm (Fig. 21.1); digital subtraction whole brain angiography (DSA) showed multiple intracranial aneurysms, basilar artery coarctation aneurysm and right AICA occlusion; basilar artery high resolution MRI imaging also showed basilar artery coarctation aneurysm, and right AICA occlusion. MRI imaging showed a basilar artery entrapment aneurysm with uneven thickness of the true lumen wall, indicating the infarction in the pontine and right pontine arm (Fig. 21.2). The patient was definitively diagnosed with a basilar artery entrapment aneurysm with acute pontine arm infarction. Stenting of the basilar artery entrapment aneurysm and subsequent treatment was performed and a good outcome was obtained. The DSA review 5 months after stenting of the basilar artery coarctation aneurysm showed a satisfactory result and no recurrence of vertigo, but no significant improvement in right ear hearing.

## 21.3 Case Review

The etiology of sudden deafness is not well understood; the two main theories are viral infection and impaired blood supply to the inner ear. Some patients with sudden deafness have a history of upper respiratory tract infection prior to the onset of the disease. The main etiology of sudden deafness with vertigo may be an impaired microcirculation in the inner ear. It is generally believed that mental stress, mood swings, irregularity in life, and sleep disorders may be the main triggers of sudden deafness. The Guidelines for the Diagnosis and Treatment of Sudden Deafness (2015) emphasize that the cause of sudden deafness is unknown and once its cause is found, an etiological diagnosis should be given, when sudden deafness is only a symptom of the associated disease and cannot be used as a diagnosis. Therefore, in this case, the patient was initially diagnosed with sudden deafness with vertigo based on the patient's symptomatic features, and the diagnosis was changed to basilar artery entrapment aneurysm with acute pontine arm infarction when the cause of sudden hearing loss was identified.

Pontine arm infarction belongs to posterior circulation infarction, and its symptoms are mostly dizziness or vertigo, deafness, tinnitus, numbness of limbs or head and face, gait or limb ataxia, and Horner syndrome. The main blood supply artery of the pontine arm comes from the (AICA) and superior cerebellar artery (SCA), and above blood supply arteries are commonly divided from the basilar artery, and the pontine arm is located in the junction area between the AICA and SCA blood supply, which is the core of the AICA innervation area and the most susceptible area to ischemia in the AICA innervation area, so the pontine arm is the diagnostic imaging marker of AICA infarction. Pontine arm infarction occurs when the main trunk of the basilar artery is narrowed or occluded. In contrast, the blood supply to the inner ear comes primarily from the basilar artery or the labyrinthine artery originating from the AICA, and the labyrinthine artery is the only terminal artery supplying the inner ear with no other peripheral collateral circulation. The labyrinthine artery directly originating from the lower basilar artery, which accounted for 13.3% of the cases, and 86.7% of the cases originated from the AICA, and the AICA mostly emanated from the labyrinthine artery outside the inner ear foramen. This patient had acute pontine arm infarction leading to hearing loss and vertigo symptoms, manifesting as an acute vestibulo-cochlear syndrome, and this pontine arm infarction was associated with basilar artery entrapment aneurysm. The patient had vertigo and hearing loss in the right ear as the main symptoms, with an acute onset and a short course, having a clear etiology and diagnosis, and by the active treatments, the patient's condition was well controlled. Firstly, not all hearing loss with vertigo can be considered as peripheral damage, and also vestibular and cochlear damages can occur in central lesions; secondly, systematic evaluation of patients with vertigo, including observation and detection of nystagmus, should be emphasized. This patient did not undergo further relevant vestibular function tests, such as head shaking nystagmus test, head impulse test, and eye movement test, because of negative spontaneous nystagmus and clear etiology. Careful bedside examination, necessary ancillary tests, and systematic evaluation of patients with vertigo can help to clarify the diagnosis, avoid misdiagnosis and underdiagnosis, and prevent life-threatening progression of the disease.

## Bibliography

Choi KD, Lee H, Kim JS. Ischemic syndromes causing dizziness and vertigo. Handb Clin Neurol. 2016;137:317–40.

Editorial Board of Chinese Journal of Otolaryngology Head and Neck Surgery, Society of Otolaryngology Head and Neck Surgery, Chinese Medical Association. Guidelines for the diagnosis and treatment of sudden deafness (2015). Chin J Otolaryngol Head Neck Surg. 2015;50(6):443–7.

Kim HA, Lee H. Recent advances in understanding audiovestibular loss of a vascular cause. J Stroke. 2017;19(1):61–6.

Newman-Toker DE. Missed stroke in acute vertigo and dizziness: it is time for action, not debate. Ann Neurol. 2016;79(1):27–31.

Venhovens J, Meulstee J, Verhagen WI. Acute vestibular syndrome: a critical review and diagnostic algorithm concerning the clinical differentiation of peripheral versus central aetiologies in the emergency department. J Neurol. 2016;263(11):2151–7.

# 22 Pontine Infarction First Diagnosed as Sudden Deafness

Jing Dai and Xizheng Shan

## 22.1 Summary of Medical Records

Patient, male, 58 years old. Complaint: Hearing loss in both ears for half a month, vertigo with numbness in the right limb for 2 days. Present history: The patient had a history of hearing loss in both ears due to the use of gentamicin, but half a month ago he felt a further hearing loss in both ears after exertion, and was diagnosed with sudden deafness at a local hospital. Two days ago, he had a sudden onset of vertigo, swaying vision, with bilateral tinnitus and ear fullness, numbness in the right limb, unsteadiness in walking with pulsion to right side, and double vision in the distance. Past history: diabetes mellitus for 6 years. Examination: spontaneous nystagmus was negative, muscle strengths of both limbs were at grade 5, muscle tones of the limbs were normal, pain and vibration sensations of the right limbs were reduced compared with the left limbs, and the right heel-knee-shin test and finger-nose test were not stable. Audiometry showed severe sensorineural deafness in both ears. Vestibular function was normal, but showing asymmetric bilateral optokinetic nystagmus, with reduced gain on both sides. Brain MRI: infarction of the left pontine near the midline (Fig. 22.1). Diagnosis: acute cerebral pontine infarction. After treatment with drugs for improving cerebral blood circulation and cerebral metabolism, nutritional nerve, anticoagulation, and lipid-lowering, the patient's right limb muscle strength basically returned to normal, without diplopia and other special complaints of discomfort, and dizziness was reduced, but hearing did not change significantly.

J. Dai
Institute of Vertigo, Third Medical Center, PLA General Hospital, Beijing, China

X. Shan (✉)
Department of Otolaryngology Head and Neck Surgery, Beijing Electric Power Teaching Hospital, Capital Medical University, Beijing, China

© Scientific and Technical Documentation Press 2023

X. Shan, E. Wang (eds.), *Interpretation of Vertigo Cases*, Experts' Perspectives on Medical Advances, https://doi.org/10.1007/978-981-99-6995-1_22

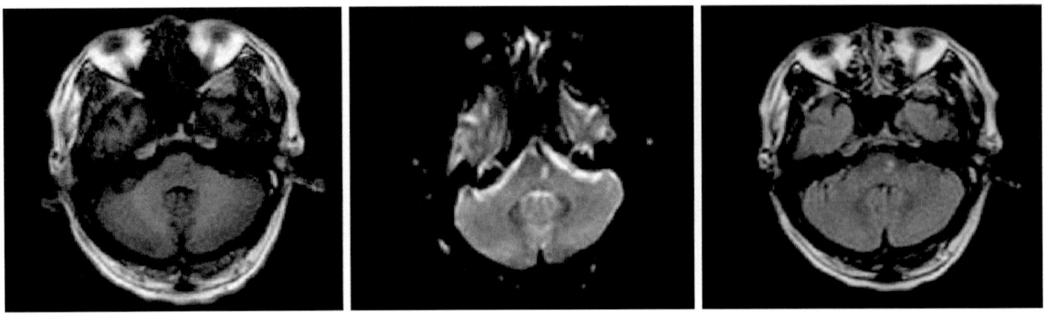

**Fig. 22.1** Brain MRI. Infarction in the left pontine near the midline, showing $T_2$ WI and DWI high signals, $T_1$ WI low signal

## 22.2 Case Study

The patient is a middle-aged male, he had previous bilateral hearing loss due to the use of gentamicin, and half a month ago the patient suddenly felt further hearing loss and was diagnosed as sudden deafness at local hospital. And 2 days ago, he developed the symptoms of vertigo, tinnitus, and ear fullness, with right-sided limb numbness, unsteady walking, right-sided pulsion, and diplopia symptoms. On examination: spontaneous nystagmus was negative, muscle strengths of both limbs were grade 5, muscle tones of the limbs were normal, pain and vibration sensations of the right limb were diminished compared with the left limb, and the right heel-knee-shin test and finger-nose test were not stable and accurate. Audiometry showed severe sensorineural deafness in both ears. Bilateral optokinetic nystagmus was asymmetric, with reduced gain on both sides. Based on the patient's symptoms, signs, and a history of diabetes mellitus for 6 years as a risk factor for stroke, the patient was considered to have the possibility of stroke. A brain MRI was performed, which showed infarction in the proximal midline of the left pontine. The patient was then definitively diagnosed with acute pontine infarction. The current Chinese guidelines for the management of sudden deafness define sudden deafness as an unexplained sensorineural hearing loss that occurs suddenly within 72 h, with a hearing loss of $\geq$20 dBHL in at least two adjacent frequencies. About 1/3 of patients with sudden deafness may have vestibular symptoms such as vertigo or dizziness and unsteadiness. It is important to note that some patients with acute cerebrovascular disease can also have sudden deafness and vertigo as their first symptoms, and their diagnosis can be easily delayed. Most patients present with only hearing loss and vertigo episodes at the first visit and are unable to distinguish at first by history and physical examination whether their symptoms are due to peripheral or central diseases, and there is a risk that acute hearing loss and vertigo episodes may also be a sign of brainstem infarction. The patient's prognosis was good due to timely management, and his right limb muscle strength returned to normal, his diplopia symptoms disappeared, and his dizziness resolved.

## 22.3 Case Review

Sudden deafness is a common disease in otology, but its etiology and pathogenesis have been controversial, and most scholars now believe that it is related to impaired blood circulation in the inner ear, so when sudden deafness is diagnosed, acute cerebral ischemia or infarction should be ruled out first. This case was able to be detected and diagnosed with pontine infarction by brain MRI. The pontine vascular supply originates from the pontine branch of the basilar artery, which is the terminal artery, and is the most common site of brainstem infarction. The internal auditory artery originates from the vertebrobasilar system, with most originating from the anterior inferior cerebellar artery and a few from the superior cerebellar artery or basilar artery.

Cerebellar peduncle or brainstem infarction caused by occlusion of the anterior inferior cerebellar artery can lead to vertigo, tinnitus, deafness on the side of the lesion, decreased or absent sensation of the side-affected face and contralateral limbs, and dysarthria and dysphonia in severe cases. The initial symptoms were hearing loss and vertigo attacks in this patient, which were due to the fact that the internal auditory artery is a terminal vessel with no collateral circulation, and the inner ear is metabolically poorly tolerant to the hypoxic environment, in addition to mechanical compression by the edematous brain tissue and involvement of the vestibulocochlear nucleus and conduction fibers located in the brainstem by infarcted foci. There may be no systemic symptoms when only presence of small vasospasms or microemboli in the absence of large vascular lesions, but as the disease progresses, patients may present with some symptoms related with cranial nerve damage such as weakness and numbness of the extremities, deviation of the corners of the mouth, and also followed by facial and limb numbness and diplopia symptoms.

Studies have showed that 25–53% of acute cerebral infarctions are associated with hypertension, diabetes, heart disease, and smoking, and that patients with these conditions are prone to spasm and clot formation in the inner ear vessels. Patients with a history of diabetes have an increased risk of stroke. Therefore, patients with such sudden deafness encountered in clinical practice should undergo relevant cardiovascular and cerebrovascular evaluation. In addition, because small focal infarcts of the cerebellum and brainstem have atypical clinical symptoms and mostly lack characteristic localizing signs, imaging is very important in addition to clinical symptoms and signs. MRI can show the infarct lesion after 4 h of ischemia, and it is the most meaningful test to diagnose brainstem infarction because of its higher resolution and sensitivity compared with CT. This patient was admitted to the hospital with sudden deafness, and the subsequent onset of symptoms was suspected to result from a stroke, which was diagnosed as acute cerebral infarction by brain MRI and was treated promptly and effectively by thrombolysis, reduction of blood viscosity, improvement of circulation, and nutrition of cerebral nerve cells increase of cerebral blood flow, reduction of ischemic neurological damage caused by vasospasm, and enhancement of energy metabolism in the brain. This patient had a better prognosis due to mild symptoms and timely treatment.

In conclusion, sudden deafness and vertigo attacks can be the prodromal or main symptoms of posterior circulation infarction, while the signs and symptoms of brain injury may not be obvious or may be delayed. In addition to systematic audiological examinations, a detailed systemic examination, brain MRI, and other ancillary examinations should be conducted according to the conditions of patient. The identification of the risk factors for cerebrovascular disease and the intervention treatments is required to reduce misdiagnosis and mismanagement.

## Bibliography

Dai XR, Zhang R, Hu JY. Two cases of posterior circulation cerebral infarction with unilateral deafness as the prodromal manifestation. Chin J Neuropsychiatr Disord. 2013;39(12):754–5.

Kim HA, Lee BC, Hong JH, et al. Long-term prognosis for hearing recovery in stroke patients presenting vertigo and acute hearing loss. J Neurol Sci. 2014;339(1-2):176–82.

# Posterior Circulation Infarction with Sudden Deafness with Vertigo as the First Symptom

23

Shujun Jiang and Ning Wang

## 23.1 Summary of Medical Records

Patient, male, 54 years old. Complaint: Sudden vertigo with hearing loss in the left ear for 3 days. Present history: The patient had sudden onset of vertigo with hearing loss in the left ear 3 days ago with no obvious cause, no nausea or vomiting, still walking independently, no impairment in body movement and sensory abnormalities, no choking or difficulty in swallowing, no symptoms of blackout or diplopia, no impairment in consciousness. Emergency head CT suggested lacunar cerebral infarction, and the patient was diagnosed as sudden deafness with vertigo, and was admitted to the hospital in emergency on January 5, 2017. Past history: having a history of hypertension, taking antihypertensive drugs irregularly, without monitoring blood pressure, no recent complaints of palpitations, chest tightness, chest pain, denied the histories of surgery and trauma, diabetes, cerebral infarction, liver disease, tuberculosis, and no history of penicillin allergy. Physical examination: body temperature 36.5 °C, pulse 80 times/min, respiratory rate 18 times/min, blood pressure 180/120 mmHg, clear consciousness, fluent speech, normal higher cortical function, bilateral pupils were normal, sensitive to light reflex, with normal eye movements, bilateral frontal lines were symmetrical, no deviation in the angle of the mouth, tongue extension was in the center position, normal for soft palate elevation, uvula was in the center, normal pharyngeal reflex, and soft neck. There was no abnormality in the heart, lungs and abdomen, no edema in the lower limbs, muscle strength was at grade 5, with moderate muscle tones, tendon reflexes were normal and symmetrical, Babinski's signs were not elicited bilaterally, pinprick sensations in the skin of the limbs were symmetrical, and no ataxic movements . Otologic examination: no abnormalities in the external auditory canal and tympanic membrane, hearing loss in the left ear, Rinne test with air conduction greater than bone conduction, Weber test with acoustic bias to the right, and negative spontaneous nystagmus. On the second day of admission, the patient showed symptoms of unsteadiness in walking, slurred speech, choking when drinking water, and numbness and weakness of the right limb. On examination: compared with the admission, blood pressure was 150/60 mmHg, with dysarthria, showing left-sided deviation of the angle of the mouth, decreased pharyngeal reflex, grade 5 for muscle strength of the right limb, positive Babinski's sign on the right side, decreased skin pinprick sensation on the right limb, ataxic movements on the left side, and no

S. Jiang
Department of Comprehensive Treatment, Second Medical Center, Chinese PLA General Hospital, Beijing, China

N. Wang (✉)
Institute of Vertigo, Electric Power Teaching Hospital, Capital Medical University, Beijing, China

© Scientific and Technical Documentation Press 2023

X. Shan, E. Wang (eds.), *Interpretation of Vertigo Cases*, Experts' Perspectives on Medical Advances, https://doi.org/10.1007/978-981-99-6995-1_23

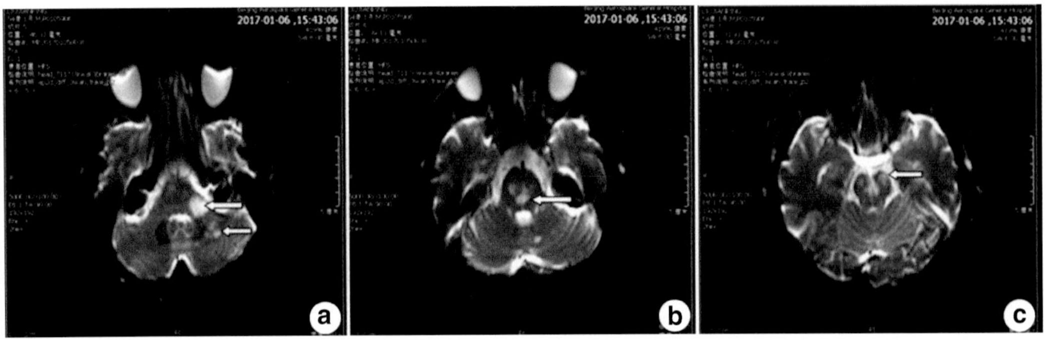


**Fig. 23.1** Brain MRI (DWI). (**a**) arrows show new infarction foci in the left cerebellum and left pontine arm; (**b**) arrow shows new infarction lesion in the pons; (**c**) shows new infarction lesion in the left cerebral peduncle

significant changes in the other signs. Otologic examination: positive horizontal and vertical gaze-induced nystagmus. Brain MRI: left cerebellum, pontine arm, pontine, cerebral peduncle, basal ganglia, and bilateral frontal areas showed multiple abnormal signals with ischemic and infarct foci, of which new lesions in the left cerebellum, pontine arm, pontine, and cerebral peduncle (Fig. 23.1). Cerebral angiography: showed slender left vertebral artery, severe stenosis of the right vertebral artery at opening, basilar artery occlusion, and incomplete opening of the posterior cerebral arteries bilaterally (Fig. 23.2). Pure tone audiometry: sensorineural deafness in the left ear. Vascular ultrasound: sclerotic plaques in the sinus of the right carotid artery and the beginning segment of the right subclavian artery. Laboratory tests: no significant abnormalities in routine blood test, approximately normal coagulation function, biochemistry test suggesting normal liver and kidney functions, TC 2.58 mmol/L, TG 0.77 mmol/L, HDL-C 0.67 mmol/L, LDL-C 1.36 mmol/L, uric acid 223.6 μmol/L, approximately normal electrolytes, negative antinuclear antibody (ANA), negative antiphospholipid antibody, and elevated serum homocysteine (44.0 μmol/L). The patient was then diagnosed with posterior circulation infarction. After admission, he was treated with drugs of antiplatelet, lipid-lowering, including aspirin 100 mg once daily, clopidogrel hydrogen sulfate 75 mg once daily, and atorvastatin 40 mg once a night. The patient was discharged with effective treatment results.

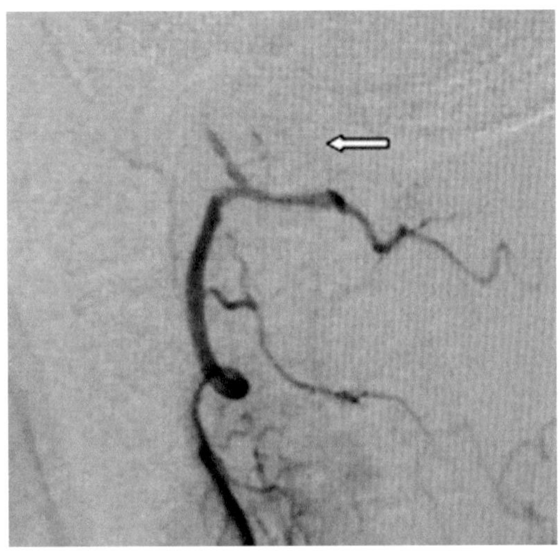

**Fig. 23.2** Cerebral angiography. The left vertebral artery was slender, the right vertebral artery near opening was severely narrowed, the basilar artery was occluded, and the posterior cerebral arteries were incompletely opened bilaterally

## 23.2 Case Study

The patient was a middle-aged male who complained of sudden dizziness with hearing loss in the left ear for 3 days without neurological symptoms such as impaired body movement, sensory abnormalities, choking on when drinking water, dysphagia, diplopia, and impaired consciousness. Emergency head CT suggested old lacunar cerebral infarction lesion, and the patient was diagnosed sudden deafness with vertigo and admitted to the hospital. The patient had a history of hypertension, but was not on regular medication and was not monitored for blood pressure, which was 180/120 mmHg on admission. Neuro-otological examination showed no other neurological abnormalities except hearing loss in the left ear, and spontaneous nystagmus was negative. However, the patient began to have neurological symptoms such as unsteadiness in walking, slurred speech, choking when drinking water, and numbness and weakness of the right limb on the fourth day after admission to the hospital. Re-examination showed that the patient had a blood pressure of 150/60 mmHg, showed dysarthria, left-sided deviation of the angle of the mouth, decreased pharyngeal reflex, grade 5 for muscle strength of the right limb, positive Babinski's sign on the right side, decreased pinprick sensation of the skin of the right limb, and ataxic movements on the left side limb. Otologic examination: emerging horizontal and vertical gaze nystagmus. Brain MRI showed multiple abnormal signals in the left cerebellum, pontine arm, pontine, cerebral peduncle, basal ganglia, and bilateral frontal areas, indicating ischemic and infarct foci, with new foci in the left cerebellum, pontine arm, pontine, and cerebral peduncle. Cerebral angiography showed slender left vertebral artery, severe stenosis of the right vertebral artery opening, basilar artery occlusion, and incomplete opening of the posterior cerebral arteries bilaterally. Pure tone audiometry showed sensorineural deafness in the left ear. Vascular ultrasound showed sclerotic spots in the sinus of the right carotid artery and the beginning of the right subclavian artery. The patient was then diagnosed with posterior circulation infarction. The patient's condition improved and stabilized after treatments with drugs of antiplatelet and lipid lowering.

## 23.3 Case Review

Sudden deafness is a common disease in otolaryngology, with incidence of 10–20/100,000. Most sudden deafness occurs in one ear, but in a few cases, both ears may be involved. About 30% of sudden deafness patients may also have vertigo symptom. The etiology of sudden deafness is not well understood. It is believed that vascular lesions are the main risk factors for this disease and the pathological mechanism of sudden deafness may be related to microthromboembolism.

In clinical practice, patients diagnosed as sudden deafness may show poor treatment outcomes or even gradual worsening of symptoms, and after complete examination and re-evaluation, it is clear that the sudden deafness is caused by acute infarction of the anterior inferior cerebellar artery (AICA). The clinical manifestations of AICA infarction are vertigo, ipsilateral tinnitus and deafness, vomiting, ipsilateral limb cerebellar ataxia, ipsilateral peripheral facial palsy, ipsilateral facial and contralateral limb and trunk pain, ipsilateral Horner's sign, and temperature disturbance. AICA infarction may involve the medulla oblongata and fibrae pyramidales. The common clinical manifestations of AICA infarction also include nystagmus. Among them, horizontal direction-changing gaze nystagmus, vertical gaze nystagmus, and torsional nystagmus (especially with direction-changing torsional nystagmus when gazing in different directions) often suggest brainstem (pontine or medulla oblongata) or cerebellar lesions. In this case, 4 days after the onset of sudden deafness, the patient presented with choking when drinking water, dysarthria, positive horizontal and vertical gaze nystagmus, left-sided sensorineural deafness, left-sided central facial palsy, decreased muscle strength in the right limb, positive Babinski's sign in the right limb, decreased skin pinprick sensation in the right limb, and ataxic movement in the left limb. The patient was diagnosed as AICA infarction in combination with brain MRI findings. The most common pathogenesis of sudden deafness due to AICA infarction is atherosclerotic thrombosis leading to inner ear ischemia, as well as the infarction of the vestibular and cochlear nerve nuclei in the pontine and their connecting fibers. Based on the characteristics of hearing damage, sudden deafness is classified as low-frequency hearing loss, high-frequency hearing loss, hearing loss with flat thresholds curve, and total deafness. High-frequency hearing loss and total deafness are highly associated with vascular injury. The presentation of AICA infarction depends on the size and location of the infarct focus. Early in the course of the disease, hearing loss may be a single symptom, and as the disease progresses, acute vestibular and auditory damages may result in ischemic damage in other parts of the posterior circulation. It is reported that some patients with AICA infarction have sudden deafness and/or vertigo as the first symptom, followed by neurological symptoms such as facial palsy appearing later in the course of the disease. The patient in this case report had episodic vertigo and sudden deafness as the first symptoms, and these cochlear and vestibular symptoms occurred before other pontocerebellar symptoms; therefore, patients with sudden deafness in the presence of multiple atherosclerotic risk factors need to be highly alert to the possibility of posterior circulation infarction. Brain MRI examination is to be performed as early as possible to avoid delay in diagnosis and treatment.

Cerebral angiography in this patient suggested the presence of basilar artery stenosis. It has been shown that 8% of patients with cerebral ischemia from basilar artery stenosis exhibit sudden deafness, which may be due to the fact that stenosis is more common in the basilar artery near the AICA opening. Patients with AICA infarction with basilar artery stenosis have decreased AICA blood flow velocity and are most likely to have ischemic injury to the inner ear, and other symptoms associated with pontocerebellar damage may occur following sudden deafness. The angle of the vertebrobasilar junction may be a risk factor for sudden deafness caused by vascular factors that damage the cochlea, and the reduced shear of blood flow on the inner surface of the vessel wall at the curvature of the vertebral artery favors atherosclerosis formation. The angled travel of the basilar artery can also cause a decrease in AICA flow velocity or accelerate AICA atherosclerosis formation. In patients with multiple risk factors, including cardiovascular disease, if presence of sudden hearing loss, especially with bilateral tinnitus, brain MRI-DWI sequences and intracranial magnetic resonance angiography (MRA) or non-traumatic angiography (CTA) should be performed to detect if presence of stenotic lesions in the lower basilar artery where AICA emanates or combined with stenotic lesions in intracranial segments of vertebral artery. Patients with sudden deafness with vertigo and other symptoms of impaired vestibular function, suspected vertebrobasilar stenosis in the cerebral vasculature, and accompanied by multiple atherosclerotic risk factors should be on high alert to avoid delaying the diagnosis and treatment of posterior circulation infarction.

## Bibliography

Choi KD, Lee H, Kim JS. Ischemic syndromes causing dizziness and vertigo. Handb Clin Neurol. 2016;137:317–40.

Halmagyi GM. Brainstem stroke preceded by transient isolated vertigo attacks. J Neurol. 2017;264(10):2170–2.

Kim HA, Lee H. Recent advances in understanding audiovestibular loss of a vascular cause. J Stroke. 2017;19(1):61–6.

# 24 Isolated Vertigo Due to Moyamoya Disease

Chunlin Zhang

## 24.1 Summary of Medical Records

Patient, female, 56 years old. Chief complaint: vertigo for 20 days. Present history: The patient had a sudden onset of severe vertigo on the way to take her grandson to school in the morning 20 days ago, and was forced to take a squatting position to hold her grandson without falling, without any impairment of consciousness, and the vertigo attack lasted for about 5 min. After returning home and resting in bed, without any obvious cause, she had another vertigo attack with rotating vision, nausea, and vomiting, not daring to open her eyes or change her position, unable to get out of bed, but no symptoms of diplopia, blackout, disfluency in speech, numbness, and weakness of the limbs, etc. She was sent to a hospital in Beijing, and was diagnosed with cerebral infarction after undergoing the examinations of head CT, brain MRI and MRA of the head and neck. Three days later, the patient's dizziness was significantly relieved and she was able to get out of bed without visual rotation, but the patient still continued to feel dizzy and unstable walking. Past history: having a history of hypertension, diabetes mellitus, and coronary heart disease. Family history: the patient's mother with a history of hypertension. The patient was admitted to hospital on October 29, 2018 for further consultation. Admission examination: good general condition, and no positive neurologic localization signs. Neurotologic examination: negative spontaneous nystagmus, and normal for the external auditory canals and tympanic membranes. Vestibular function examination: faint rightward horizontal spontaneous nystagmus was seen with a slow phase velocity of 2°/s. Positional tests: lying-down test, roll test and Dix-Hallpike test were negative. Velocity step test: normal and symmetrical post-rotational nystagmus (CP = 3.5%). Caloric test showed normal and symmetrical functions of bilateral horizontal semicircular canals (CP = 5%). Visual dysmetria test was normal bilaterally. Visual smooth pursuit test showed type II curve. No abnormality in the optokinetic nystagmus test. Negative head-shaking nystagmus. Posturography: static posture chart (eyes open) with anterior-posterior center of gravity, total trajectory length of 28.2 cm; static posture chart (eyes closed) with anterior-posterior center of gravity, total trajectory length of 28.4 cm; sponge pad (eyes open) with central distribution of center of gravity, total trajectory length of about 35.1 cm; and sponge pad (eyes closed) with central distribution, total trajectory length of 56.3 cm. Pure tone audiometry: hearing was basically normal in both ears. Tympanography: both tympanograms showed type-A curves. Stapedial muscle acoustic reflex: elicited at all frequencies in the right ear, not elicited at 2 and 4 kHz in the left ear. No abnor-

C. Zhang (✉)
Department of Neurology, Central Hospital of Liuzhou Railway, Liuzhou, China

© Scientific and Technical Documentation Press 2023
X. Shan, E. Wang (eds.), *Interpretation of Vertigo Cases*, Experts' Perspectives on Medical Advances, https://doi.org/10.1007/978-981-99-6995-1_24

malities were found in auditory brainstem response (ABR) testing. Cervical vestibular evoked myogenic potentials (c-VEMP): bilateral asymmetry ratio 1.6, $P_1$ latency 21.8 ms, $N_1$ latency 30.7 ms, $P_1$–$N_1$ amplitude 97.7 μV in the left ear; $P_1$ latency 21.7 ms, $N_1$ latency 31.5 ms, $P_1$–$N_1$ amplitude 100.8 μV in the right ear. Thirty-two points on the anxiety self-rating scale and 36 points on the depression self-rating scale. After admission, secondary prevention treatment of cerebrovascular disease was continued, and Ginkgo biloba extract injection and other drugs to improve blood circulation were given. After treatment, the patient's symptoms of dizziness and unsteady walking were completely resolved. With neurological and neurosurgical consultations and previous head and neck MRA findings, the moyamoya disease was considered and then brain magnetic resonance perfusion imaging was performed, indicating the reduced perfusion in the bilateral parietal-temporal lobes (Fig. 24.1). The following whole brain angiography (DSA) showed the typical signs of cerebral moyamoya disease (Fig. 24.2). The patient was then diag-

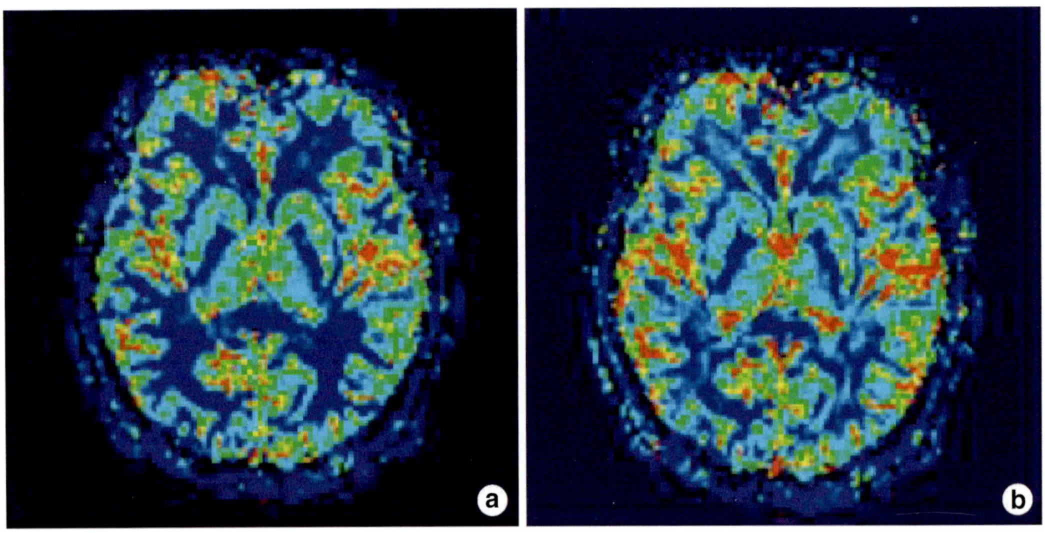


**Fig. 24.1** Brain magnetic resonance perfusion imaging. (**a**) Cerebral blood flow; (**b**) cerebral blood volume

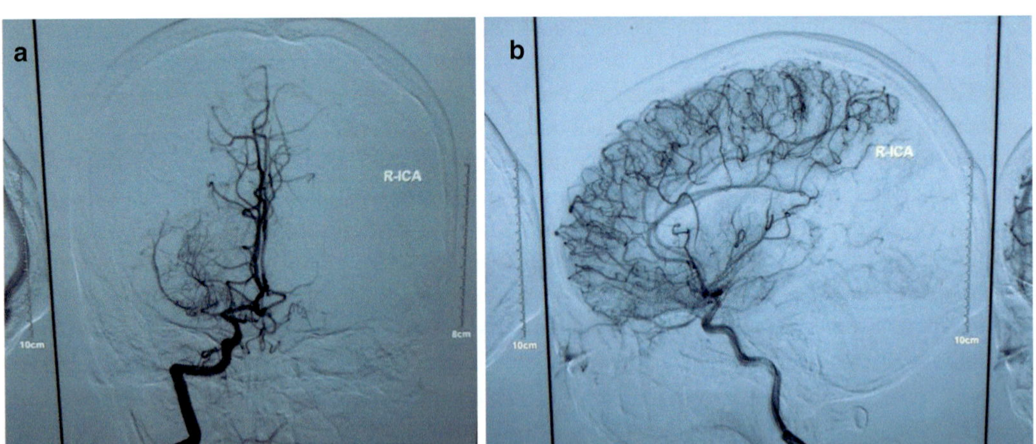


**Fig. 24.2** Right internal carotid artery angiography. (**a**) Anterior-posterior view; (**b**) lateral view

nosed with moyamoya disease and discharged from the hospital. The patient was treated according to the secondary prevention protocol for cerebrovascular disease and was instructed to repeat brain MRI and CTA (or DSA) 6 months after discharge.

## 24.2 Case Study

Vestibular vertigo is classified into central vertigo and peripheral vertigo according to the sites of the lesions. The vestibular center includes the vestibular nucleus, the vestibular pathway in the brainstem, the base of the fourth ventricle and adjacent structures (flocculonodular lobe and inferior cerebellar vermis), the posterior lateral nucleus of the thalamus, the vestibulo-spinal pathway, and the vestibular cortex of the brain. Lesions of these central vestibular structures cause asymmetry in bilateral vestibular functions, resulting in vertigo or dizziness. Typical central vertigo is often combined with localized neurological symptoms and signs, such as diplopia, dysarthria, dysphagia, hemiparesis, ataxia, and others, and is usually not difficult to diagnose. Isolated vertigo is a type of vertigo that is not associated with other localized neurological symptoms and signs, and it is often difficult to distinguish between central and peripheral vestibular lesions. The common causes of central isolated vertigo are cerebrovascular diseases (posterior circulation transient ischemic attack, cerebral infarction, cerebral hemorrhage), brain tumors, multiple sclerosis, and genetic and degenerative diseases. Isolated vertigo can be the only manifestation of acute cerebrovascular disease, and early and timely recognition of isolated vertigo due to acute vascular diseases (stroke) is very important to reduce the serious consequences of these diseases. In addition to detailed bedside examinations and vestibular function tests, a thorough assessment of risk factors for cerebrovascular diseases and brain imaging (including cerebrovascular imaging) should be performed timely in patients with acute isolated vertigo. Common risk factors for cerebrovascular disease are as follows. (1) Age > 50 years. (2) Blood pressure > 140/90 mmHg, which is high risk. (3) Cardiovascular disease, such as coronary artery disease, hypertension, and atrial fibrillation. (4) Hyperlipidemia and hypercholesterolemia, with LDL:HDL in the range of 130–159 as intermediate risk and a ratio > 160 as high risk. (5) Diabetes mellitus. (6) Stroke, white matter lesions, cerebrovascular disease. (7) Smoking. (8) Overweight. (9) Tension-stress-anxiety. (10) A sedentary-resting lifestyle. (11) Family history of high risks, such as hypertension, heart disease, stroke, diabetes. Isolated vertigo with more than three of these risk factors should be highly suspicious for transient ischemic attack (TIA) or stroke and secondary prevention of cerebrovascular disease is recommended. In this case, the patient was a female with hypertension, diabetes mellitus, coronary artery disease, and her mother had a history of hypertension, with more than three risk factors. At the initial diagnosis, no significant abnormality was seen on the brain MRI at the hospital, bilateral middle cerebral artery stenosis with abundant collateral circulation compensation was seen on head and neck MRA, and the possibility of moyamoya disease was considered. And also the vestibular function and audiological examination did not support the diagnosis of peripheral vertigo. Following brain magnetic resonance perfusion imaging suggested bilateral parietal-temporal lobe hypoperfusion, and whole brain angiography confirmed the diagnosis of moyamoya disease. The patient was treated with secondary prevention protocol for cerebrovascular disease, including aspirin combined with clopidogrel bisulfate antiplatelet and atorvastatin, with a good treatment outcome. No stroke lesion was seen on brain MRI at the beginning and more than 20 days after the onset of the illness, but the clinical findings and treatment results of other two hospitals indicated the diagnosis of cerebral infarction, therefore the clinical consideration of cerebral infarction due to moyamoya disease remained. The Chinese Expert Consensus on the Diagnosis and Treatment of Moyamoya Disease and Moyamoya Syndrome (2017) recommends the timing of surgery and non-surgical treatment as follows: there is no clear evidence on the timing of surgery, although general evidence supports that the earlier cerebral revascularization surgery is performed after the diagnosis is confirmed, the better the patient's outcome is. However, it is sometimes reasonable to delay surgery, such as with a recent history of cerebral infarction, infection, or bleeding. Aggressive pharmacological treatment of the underlying or concomitant disease is recommended. Management of risk factors for stroke and lifestyle guidance should complement each other. In this case of ischemic moyamoya disease, the patient initially presented with symptoms of reversible neurological deficit, with well-compensated collateral circulation as seen on DSA, we refer to the recommendations of the expert consensus on treatment strategy for moyamoya disease and withhold revascularization surgery.

## 24.3 Case Review

Central vertigo accounts for a minority of cases of dizziness or vertigo, but it is harmful and sometimes malignant. Early screening of central vertigo from patients with isolated vertigo is currently a difficult problem and also one of the most important problems to be dealt with actively. The present case is a successful management of isolated vertigo. Brain MRI (including DWI sequences) is far more sensitive than CT for cerebral infarcts (especially brainstem and cerebellar infarcts), but various authors have reported a percentage of false-negative rates early in the onset (ranging from 24 h to 1 week). Therefore, in patients with isolated vertigo with suspected stroke, a first negative brain MRI early in the onset still cannot completely exclude stroke, and brain MRI should be repeated at an appropriate time, and if necessary, brain thin-section scanning and whole-brain angiography should be performed to assist in the diagnosis of the cause of vertigo. Central vasogenic vertigo is mostly caused by vascular lesions in the posterior circulation. In this case, DSA suggested moyamoya disease, cerebral vascular lesions in the anterior circulation, and combined with the reduced perfusion in the parieto-temporal lobe as seen with brain magnetic resonance perfusion imaging. Vertigo may be caused by ischemia in the anterior circulation affecting the temporoparietal vestibular cortex.

## Bibliography

Choi KH, Lee SH, Kim JM, et al. Rotational vertebral artery syndrome in moyamoya disease: a sign of unilateral vertebral artery stenosis. Clin Neurol Neurosurg. 2013;115(9):1900–2.

Fujimura M, Bang OY, Kim JS. Moyamoya disease. Front Neurol Neurosci. 2016;40:204–20.

Hishikawa T, Sugiu K, Date I. Moyamoya disease: a review of clinical research. Acta Med Okayama. 2016;70(4):229–36.

Kim H, Jang DK, Han YM, et al. Direct bypass versus indirect bypass in adult moyamoya angiopathy with symptoms or hemodynamic instability: a meta-analysis of comparative studies. World Neurosurg. 2016;94:273–84.

Zhang H, Zheng L, Feng L. Epidemiology, diagnosis and treatment of moyamoya disease (review). Exp Ther Med. 2019;17(3):1977–84.

# 25 Vertigo Due to Vertebrobasilar Dolichoectasia

Xuetao Mu

## 25.1 Summary of Medical Records

Patient, male, 60 years old. Complaint: Recurrent episodes of vertigo for 6 years and one episode of blackout. Present history: The patient has recurrent episodes of vertigo, mostly rotational, of variable duration for the past 6 years, without significant hearing loss, tinnitus, or headache, except for symptoms with nausea. Past history: history of renal transplantation and previous brain MRI suggesting multiple lacunar infarct foci in the brain. Physical examination: no positive signs on otologic and neurologic examination. Brain MRA and diagnosis: vertebrobasilar dolichoectasia (VBD) (Fig. 25.1).

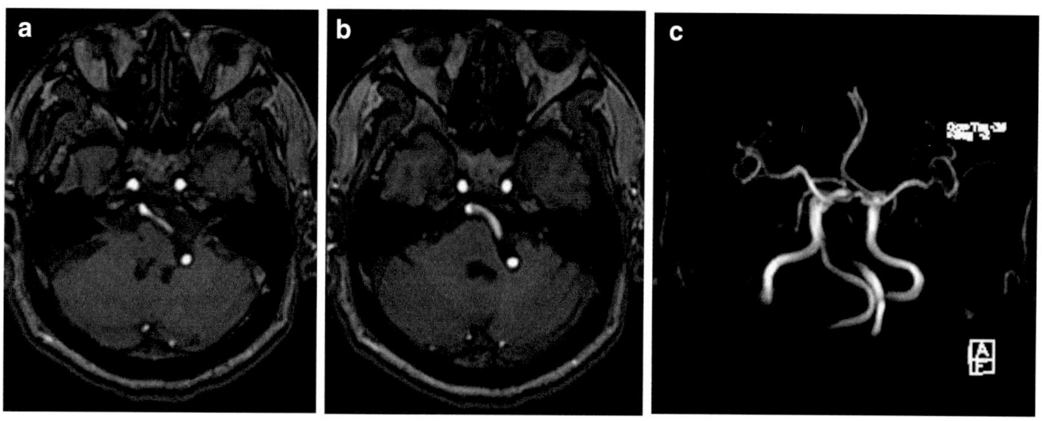

**Fig. 25.1** Brain MRA. Three-dimensional time-of-flight (3D-TOF) images show the right vertebral artery riding across to the left with a grade 3 offset and significant brainstem compression (**a**, **b**). Maximum density projection (MIP) image: shows a length of >23.5 mm of the intracranial segment of the vertebral artery with a lateral deviation of >10 mm from the vertical line between the entrance of the intracranial segment of the vertebral artery to the origin of the basilar artery (**c**)

X. Mu (✉)
Department of Magnetic Resonance Imaging, Third Medical Center, PLA General Hospital, Beijing, China

© Scientific and Technical Documentation Press 2023
X. Shan, E. Wang (eds.), *Interpretation of Vertigo Cases*, Experts' Perspectives on Medical Advances, https://doi.org/10.1007/978-981-99-6995-1_25

## 25.2 Case Study

Prolonged dilatation of the vertebral basilar artery was first proposed by Smoker et al. in 1986 and refers to abnormal tortuosity, dilatation, and lengthening of the vertebral basilar artery. The incidence of the disease ranges from 0.06% to 5.8% in the general population and up to 10% to 12% in stroke patients. The etiology of vertebrobasilar artery prolonged dilatation is unknown, and the likely pathophysiological mechanism is based on congenital defects of the intravascular elastic membrane and muscular layer, under the influence of hypertension, diabetes mellitus, and vascular sclerosis, associated with abnormal vascular remodeling or abnormal connective tissue of the arterial wall due to an imbalance between matrix metalloproteinase and antiproteinase activities in the connective tissue. Based on clinical manifestations, prolonged dilatation of the vertebrobasilar artery can be classified as follows: (1) Asymptomatic type: most cases have this type, accounting for 70%. (2) Posterior circulation ischemic type: it may manifest with symptoms of vertigo attacks, visual rotation with blurred vision, tinnitus, etc., infarction in the posterior cerebral circulation blood supply area, ipsilateral cerebral nerve palsy with motor and sensory dysfunction of the contralateral limb, or bilateral limb motor and sensory dysfunction, or bilateral ocular coordination dysfunction and cerebellar dysfunction, etc. It has been suggested that prolonged dilatation of the vertebrobasilar artery is a cause of cerebral infarction independent of vascular risk factors such as age, hypertension, and diabetes mellitus. In addition, hemorrhagic strokes caused by prolonged dilatation of the vertebral basilar artery are not uncommon. (3) Brainstem compression type: The prolonged dilated artery produces direct compression of the brainstem. The vestibular nucleus is located at the junction of the pons and medulla oblongata, and a tortuous and thick vertebrobasilar artery can compress the part of the brainstem, which can compress the vestibular nucleus and vestibular pathways, thus causing vertigo, and the symptoms in this case are mainly caused by brainstem compression. (4) Vascular-neural syndrome type: tortuous and dilated vessels compress the adjacent nerves, often involving the VII, V, and VIII pairs of cerebral nerves. (5) Hemorrhage type: mostly related to the rupture of the entrapped aneurysm. (6) Hydrocephalus type.

The diagnosis of prolonged dilatation of the vertebrobasilar artery is based primarily on imaging. The diagnostic criteria for cranial CT angiography (CTA) are as follows: (1) Graded on the basis of the length of the dorsum of the saddle, the suprasellar pool and the third ventricle as boundaries. Grade 0, below or at the same level as the dorsum of the saddle; grade 1, below or at the same level as the suprasellar pool; grade 2, located between the suprasellar pool and the base of the third ventricle; and grade 3, at or above the level of the third ventricle. (2) Grading was performed on the degree of offset using the dorsal and slope of the saddle, the paramedian, the rim and beyond the rim, or the pontocerebellar angle. Grade 0, the midline of the basilar artery lies in the midline of the dorsal or slope of the saddle; grade 1, between the midline of the slope or saddle and the paramedian; grade 2, between the paramedian and the slope, the rim of the saddle; and grade 3, outside the rim of the dorsal and slope or reaching the pontocerebellar angle pool. (3) Prolonged dilatation of the vertebral basilar artery was defined if the height was ≥grade 2 or the offset was ≥grade 2 and the diameter was ≥4.5 mm. Semi-quantitative diagnostic criteria for MRA: the length of the basilar artery >29.5 mm and lateral deviation of >10 mm from the vertical line between the origin and the apex of the basilar artery were determined as abnormal; the length of the intracranial segment of the vertebral artery >23.5 mm and lateral deviation of >10 mm from the vertical line between the entrance to the intracranial segment of the vertebral artery and the origin of the basilar artery were determined as abnormal. DSA is a gold standard for the diagnosis of prolonged dilatation of the vertebrobasilar artery, but its use is limited by its invasiveness and inability to visualize the relationship between the vessel and brain tissue. Asymptomatic patients with prolonged dilatation of the vertebral basilar artery may be left untreated, and patients with ischemic stroke should be treated with antithrombotic therapy for atherosclerosis. Surgical treatment is the main option for compression caused by prolonged dilatation of the basilar artery, including microvascular decompression and repositioning, endoluminal revascularization, aneurysm clamping, and endovascular stenting.

## 25.3 Case Review

Elderly patients with vertigo are often diagnosed with posterior circulation ischemia on the basis of slowed blood flow on transcranial Doppler ultrasound, however, some symptoms of posterior circulation ischemia may simply be a manifestation of prolonged dilatation of the vertebral basilar artery. In this case, the slowing of blood flow in the vertebral basilar artery with prolonged dilatation resulted in inadequate blood supply to the distal microvessels, causing the development of posterior circulation ischemic vertigo; the slow blood flow predisposed the vessel walls to the formation of appendage thrombi, aggravating atherosclerosis; when prolonged dilatation of the vertebral basilar artery occurred, the basilar artery located in the basal sulcus deviated in its course, resulting in compression of the microvessels on the surface of the pontine, causing impaired blood flow distorting the prolonged basilar artery will push and produce ventral pressure traces on the pontine, directly compressing the brainstem nuclei and developing neurological dysfunction in the corresponding nuclei. Normally, the natural history of prolonged dilatation of the basilar artery is slow, however, once the disease progresses, the risk of hemorrhagic or ischemic stroke is significantly higher and the mortality rate is significantly higher than in patients with compression symptoms alone or asymptomatic patients. The early identification of the symptom-prone prolonged dilation of the vertebral basilar artery can facilitate early primary prevention of cerebral vascular diseases, and strict blood pressure control may help to reduce the incidence of symptoms (especially vascular symptoms).

## Bibliography


Chen B, Liu YF, Ren B. Clinical and imaging analysis of prolonged dilatation of the vertebral basilar artery. J Brain Neurol Disord. 2017;25(11):681–4.

Gibow RC, Ruhl DS, Hashisaki GT, et al. Unilateral sensorineural hearing loss associated with vertebrobasilar dolichoectasia. Otol Neurotol. 2018;39(1):e56–7.

Li JW, Xiang SS, Ling F, et al. A case of prolonged dilatation of the vertebral basilar artery with basilar artery entrapment aneurysm causing subarachnoid space hemorrhage. Chin J Modern Neurol Dis. 2016;16(12):845–9.

Yuan YJ, Xu K, Luo Q, Yu JL. Research progress on vertebrobasilar dolichoectasia. Int J Med Sci. 2014;11(10):1039–48.

# 26 Bickerstaff Brainstem Encephalitis with Vertigo as the Main Complaint

Qing Sun

## 26.1 Summary of Medical Records

Patient, female, 72 years old. Chief complaint: vertigo for 24 days. Present history: The patient began to experience vertigo 24 days ago. The vertigo persisted and worsened with activity and was accompanied by unstable walking, swaying vision, diplopia, nausea and vomiting, no change in hearing, clear speech, no headache, impaired consciousness, dysphagia, limb numbness, and impaired movement. The patient reported that before the onset of vertigo, she had visited the local hospital with a cold and fever, and her body temperature reached 39.5 °C. Later, her symptoms gradually decreased, but dizziness persisted, and visual stimulation could aggravate the symptoms of dizziness and unstable walking. The patient was admitted to the hospital for further treatment after more than 3 weeks of onset. Examination: clear consciousness, fluent speech, no facial palsy, negative spontaneous nystagmus, active eye movements with difficulty in fixation, hyperalgesia and hypotonia of limbs, less stable and accurate for bilateral finger-nose tests and heel-knee-shin tests, active tendon reflexes, positive perioral reflexes, and bilateral Babinski's signs. Other neurological examinations showed no abnormalities. Audiological examination: moderate sensorineural deafness in both ears. Vestibular function examination: negative spontaneous nystagmus, negative position test, hyperfunction of bilateral horizontal semicircular canals on caloric tests. Brain MRI: ischemia foci in the subcortex of the left frontal lobe and next to the left posterior horn of the lateral ventricle; hyaline septal cavity; and senile brain changes. Cerebrospinal fluid examination: pressure 115/70 $mmH_2O$, leukocytes $6 \times 10^6/L$, protein 1.197 g/L. Diagnosis: Bickerstaff brainstem encephalitis. The patient was treated with immunoglobulin and hormones, and she was discharged in good condition.

## 26.2 Case Study

Bickerstaff brainstem encephalitis is an inflammatory disease of the brainstem and manifests clinically as acute symmetric extraocular muscle paralysis, ataxia, accompanied by impaired consciousness and/or pyramidal fasciculus signs. The etiology and pathogenesis of the disease are unclear and may be related to viral infection or inflammatory demyelinating changes. It is not easily diagnosed clinically, and other central disorders need to be excluded; those with vertigo as the main complaint also need to be differentiated from peripheral vertigo disorders. In this case, the patient had a history of upper respiratory tract infection before the onset of the disease, and the

Q. Sun (✉)
Institute of Vertigo, Third Medical Center, PLA General Hospital, Beijing, China

© Scientific and Technical Documentation Press 2023

X. Shan, E. Wang (eds.), *Interpretation of Vertigo Cases*, Experts' Perspectives on Medical Advances, https://doi.org/10.1007/978-981-99-6995-1_26

main manifestations were vertigo and unsteadiness in standing and walking. Bilateral finger-nose tests and heel-knee-tibial tests were not stable and accurate, suggesting bilateral ataxia. Bilateral Babinski's signs and bilateral pyramidal tract signs were positive, and diplopia was present during the course of the disease, suggesting damage to the oculomotor nerve. The ataxia, pyramidal tract sign, and oculomotor nerve injury lesions were localized to the brainstem. Simultaneous glove-like and sock-like hypesthesia and hypotonia of the extremities suggested peripheral nerve involvement. The simultaneous involvement of the peripheral and central nervous systems was consistent with the diagnosis of a variant of Guillain-Barre syndrome. The patient had a history of upper respiratory tract infection before the onset of the disease, with an acute onset and a long duration (24 days), and her symptoms gradually resolved. With brain MRI examination, new infarct foci and occupying lesions in the brainstem were excluded, and the lumbar puncture cerebrospinal fluid examination showed the protein cell separation phenomenon, suggesting inflammatory lesions. Due to the current limitations of anti-GQ1b antibody IgG testing in China, the patient was not able to undergo such antibody testing. However, the patient's diagnosis was consistent with Bickerstaff brainstem encephalitis based on the localized and qualitative diagnostic findings. The improvement of patient's condition after treatments with immunoglobulin and hormone was also consistent with the diagnosis of inflammatory demyelinating disease.

## 26.3 Case Review

Bickerstaff brainstem encephalitis has a predominantly central nervous system involvement, mainly involving the midbrain, pons, medulla oblongata, and basal ganglia, but may also be associated with peripheral nervous system lesions. This disease often has an acute or subacute clinical onset, with most patients having symptoms of prodromal infection, commonly upper respiratory tract infection, and may present with symmetrical ocular muscle palsy, ataxia, consciousness disorder such as drowsiness and coma, hyperreflexia, and positive pathological signs and pupillary abnormalities. The cause of Bickerstaff brainstem encephalitis is unknown, but it is now believed to be an autoimmune disease caused by an immune response induced by certain inflammatory pathogenic factors, resulting in the production of anti-GQ1b antibodies. GQ1b is an autoimmune disease caused by anti-GQ1b antibodies to the extramedullary portion of the brain nerves and the neuromuscular junction, the muscle spindle, class Ia muscle afferent nerve fibers and the dorsal root ganglion of the peripheral nervous system, and the brainstem in humans. It was found that specific anti-GQ1b antibody IgG was prevalent in the sera of patients with Bickerstaff brainstem encephalitis.

Many central disorders can have vertigo, dizziness, or balance disturbances as their primary manifestation, and central nervous system lesions can easily be overlooked if the patient has relatively mild CNS manifestations and does not present with impaired consciousness or hemiparesis. Therefore, history taking and physical examination are crucial. Acute vestibular syndrome is commonly seen in peripheral vestibular disorders, which is most often seen in vestibular neuritis, sudden deafness with vertigo, labyrinthitis, and Hunt's syndrome. Acute vestibular syndrome can also be seen in central disorders, which is commonly seen in ischemic infarction of the posterior circulation. This patient with Bickerstaff brainstem encephalitis mainly presented with persistent vertigo and unsteadiness in standing and walking, with no abnormal brain MRI findings, which could easily be misdiagnosed as peripheral vertigo disease if detailed history taking and physical examination were not performed. The patient's accompanying signs of central neuropathy helped to differentiate this disease from peripheral vertigo. Early diagnosis and timely treatment of Bickerstaff brainstem encephalitis is expected to result in a better prognosis.

## Bibliography

Chen PR, Chen SP. Posterior reversible encephalopathy as the first manifestation of Bickerstaff's brainstem encephalitis. BMC Neurol. 2016;16(1):215.

Feng J, Fu X, Xie W, et al. A case report of overlapping Bickerstaff brainstem encephalitis and Guillain-Barre syndrome. Neuro Endocrinol Lett. 2013;34(7):601–5.

Fong CY, Aung HW, Khairani A, et al. Bickerstaff's brainstem encephalitis with overlapping Guillain-Barre syndrome: usefulness of sequential nerve conduction studies. Brain and Development. 2018;40(6):507–11.

Jing C, Wang Z, Chu C, et al. Miller-Fisher syndrome complicated by Bickerstaff brainstem encephalitis: a case report. Medicine. 2018;97(9):e9824.

Kundu GK, Rahman MM, Paul BK, et al. Bickerstaff's brainstem encephalitis-a case report. Mymensingh Med J. 2015;24(3):628–30.

# 27 Vertigo Due to Basilar Invagination

Xuetao Mu

## 27.1 Summary of Medical Records

Patient, female, 80 years old. Complaint: Paroxysmal vertigo for 5 years, progressive aggravation with chest discomfort for 2 years. Present history: The patient has had recurrent episodes of vertigo in the past 5 years, and her episodes of vertigo have been progressively aggravated with chest tightness and discomfort for the past 2 years, without symptoms of hearing loss or tinnitus. On cranial MRI, she was diagnosed with basilar invagination and multiple lacunar infarct foci in the brain (Fig. 27.1).

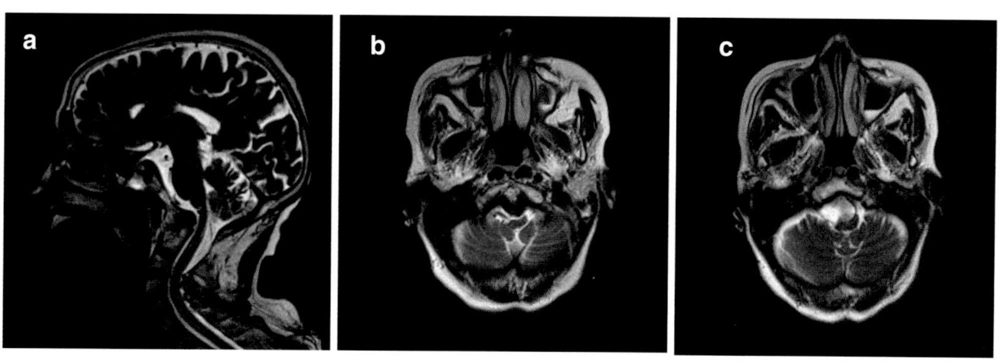


**Fig. 27.1** Cranial MRI. $T_2$ WI shows superior displacement of the dentate process of the cardinal vertebrae with significant compression of the medulla oblongata and upper cervical medulla ventralis and compression of the right vertebral artery. (**a**) Sagittal view; (**b, c**) axial view

X. Mu (✉)
Department of Magnetic Resonance Imaging, Third Medical Center, PLA General Hospital, Beijing, China

© Scientific and Technical Documentation Press 2023
X. Shan, E. Wang (eds.), *Interpretation of Vertigo Cases*, Experts' Perspectives on Medical Advances, https://doi.org/10.1007/978-981-99-6995-1_27

## 27.2 Case Study

The patient is an elderly female who complained of recurrent episodes of vertigo over the last 5 years, and her vertigo symptoms have worsened over the last 2 years. The cranial MRI showed typical basilar invagination with significant compression of the medulla oblongata and upper cervical medulla and compression of the right vertebral artery. Therefore, the patient was clearly diagnosed with basilar invagination. The patient's vertigo symptoms may be related to the inadequate blood supply to the vertebrobasilar artery caused by the basilar invagination. Patients with symptomatic basilar invagination, combined with atlantoaxial subluxation, should be operated on as soon as possible to reset or grind down the dentate process to completely relieve the compression on nerves and stabilize the atlantoaxial joint. In this case, the patient was not treated surgically because of the absence of subungual herniation and atlantoaxial subluxation, and also because of her age.

## 27.3 Case Review

Basilar invagination, also known as skull base entrapment, is caused by various types of abnormal development at the craniocervical junction during the developmental stage of the body, resulting in flattening, inversion, and entrapment of the skull base, which in turn causes compression of the brainstem, spinal cord, and other nerves, eventually forming various neurological neurospinal syndromes. Patients with basilar invagination tend to develop symptoms after youth and progress slowly, and clinical symptoms may be triggered or aggravated by sudden head force. It is often accompanied by short neck, webbed neck, low posterior hairline, posterior neck pain, head and neck immobility, forced head position and short stature, and other special appearance. Basilar invagination is divided into two phases according to the presence or absence of symptoms, the first phase is asymptomatic and the second phase is symptomatic. Also, basilar invagination can be divided into six types, namely, high cervical medullary, cerebellar, hydrocephalic, basilar artery, posterior group cranial nerve, and mixed. In addition, basilar invagination can be classified into type I and type II according to whether it is combined with a submicrocephalic tonsillar herniation malformation or classified into types A and B according to whether it was combined with atlantoaxial subluxation or not.

In the past, the diagnosis of basilar invagination was mainly based on X-ray plain radiographs. The application of thin-layer CT and MRI has greatly improved the accuracy of the diagnosis of craniocervical commissures, and thus they are widely used in the diagnosis of basilar invagination. The Chamberlain line, McGregor line, and McRae line are usually used as marker lines to evaluate and diagnose basilar invagination. On the sagittal thin-section CT bone window, basilar invagination is diagnosed when the dentate process exceeds 3 mm above the Chamberlain line, or the connecting line between the posterior border of the hard palate and the posterior border of the greater occipital foramen. In the median sagittal view, the posterior margin of the hard palate and the posterior margin of the foramen magnum were clearly identifiable, so the McGregor and McRae lines did not need to be double-counted. In the transverse axial dentate level, atlantoaxial subluxation is present when the atlanto-dental spacing (the distance between the posterior edge of the anterior atlantoaxial arch and the anterior edge of the pontine dentate) is greater than 3 mm; when the atlanto-dental spacing is less than 3 mm, there is no atlantoaxial subluxation, and the dentate subluxation is caused by a flattened skull base, i.e., the angle between the line from the nasal root to the center of the pterygoid saddle and the line from the center of the pterygoid saddle to the anterior edge of the foramen magnum (skull base angle) is greater than 145°. MRI sagittal imaging plays a crucial role in clinical diagnosis and management of the disease by determining the bony structural abnormalities and evaluating whether there is a combination of submicrocephalic tonsillar herniation deformity, spinal cord cavitation, and compression of the ventral aspect of the medulla oblongata.

It is still controversial whether surgery should be performed in patients with asymptomatic basilar invagination. The main procedures used in the treatment of basilar invagination, combined with atlantoaxial subluxation, include suboccipital decompression plus occipitocervical fusion internal fixation via the posterior approach, atlantoaxial repositioning plus fusion internal fixation, transoral dentatectomy plus repositioning fixation, transoral atlantoaxial subluxation release plus repositioning fixation, and dentatectomy via the distal lateral approach to the occipital neck or the posterior lateral approach to the suboccipital region.

## Bibliography


Salunke P, Sahoo S, Deepak AN. Different facets in management of congenital atlantoaxial dislocation and basilar invagination. Neurosurgery. 2015;77(6):e985–7.

Xia H, Yin QS, Ai FZ, et al. Treatment of basilar invagination with at lantoaxial dislocation: at lantoaxial joint distraction and fixation with transoral at lantoaxial reduction plate (TARP) without odontoidectomy. Eur Spine J. 2014;23(8):1648–55.

Yang H, Zhong S, Hu Y, et al. Rotational vertebral artery occlusion in a patient with basilar invagination. Br J Neurosurg. 2019;17:1–3.

# 28 Wernicke's Encephalopathy

Yuanxing Chen

## 28.1 Summary of Medical Records

Patient, male, 43 years old. Complaint: dizziness for more than 20 days, aggravated for 1 week. Present history: The patient began to experience transient dizziness 20 days ago when climbing a slope or going upstairs, with a sense of intoxication and no sense of rotation of visual objects. The dizziness lasted for 2–3 min, so he was seen at a local hospital, where a head CT examination showed no significant abnormalities. After 1 week of treatment, the patient's dizziness was not relieved and continued to worsen, especially when he turned his head, and he began to experience unstable walking, and his symptoms worsened when climbing hills and stairs, but his daily life was not yet significantly affected. Afterwards, the patient's condition continued to worsen progressively, the patient felt that his body swayed back and forth, and his symptoms worsened when he moved or changed position, and that the symptoms could be relieved after a few minutes of rest in a sitting or lying position. Half a month later, he developed further symptoms such as trembling vision, fear of opening eyes, repeated vomiting, and stumbling in walking. Past history: The patient had a history of chronic gastritis for more than 10 years and had not been treated systematically. On examination: clear consciousness, fluent speech, with normal abilities in memory, comprehension, and calculation, presenting with eye clonus and blurred vision, bilateral limb muscle strength at grade 5, normal muscle tone, finger-nose test and heel-knee-shin test, bilateral limb tendon reflexes (++), bilateral Babinski's signs (−). After admission, the patient was treated with medication to improve microcirculation and nerve nutrition, including glucocorticoids, anti-dizziness and antiemetic drugs, but the clinical symptoms did not improve and further worsened, and symptoms such as speech dysfluency and body tremors appeared, the body tremors started in the shoulders, gradually developed to the head, increased after activity, and gradually improved after resting. Re-examination: still having clear consciousness, certain abilities in memory, comprehension and calculation, but speech dysfluency, eye clonus, blurred vision, involuntary movements of the head and neck, bilateral limb muscle strength at grade 5, normal muscle tone, bilateral finger-nose tests were stable and accurate, but bilateral heel-knee-shin tests were not stable and accurate, bilateral limb tendon reflexes (++), and bilateral Babinski's signs (+). Ancillary tests: serum folate level 3.56 nmol/L; vitamin $B_{12}$ level 50 pmol/L; autoantibody profile ANA was weakly positive; thyroid hormone tests showed no significant abnormalities.

Y. Chen (✉)
Institute of Vertigo, Third Medical Center, PLA General Hospital, Beijing, China

© Scientific and Technical Documentation Press 2023
X. Shan, E. Wang (eds.), *Interpretation of Vertigo Cases*, Experts' Perspectives on Medical Advances, https://doi.org/10.1007/978-981-99-6995-1_28

Cerebrospinal fluid examination: colorless and clear, total number of cells was 5, protein qualitative test negative, and protein concentration 0.47 g/L. Cerebrospinal fluid viral antibody tests: negative for herpes monocytogenes virus type I IgM antibody, coxsackie group A and B virus IgM antibody, cytomegalovirus IgM antibody, rubella virus IgM antibody, measles virus IgM antibody, ECHO virus IgM antibody, and EBV IgA/VCA, IgA/EA, IgM/VCA, and IgG/VCA antibodies, and also negative for anti-Hu, anti-Ri and anti-Yo antibodies. Serum anti-Hu and anti-Ri antibodies were negative, and anti-Yo antibodies were weakly positive. Brain MRI: showing no significant abnormalities. The patient was considered to be suffering from Wernicke's encephalopathy, and treated with drugs, including glucocorticoid, drugs for improving microcirculatory, and vitamin supplementation. The patient was discharged from the hospital with improvement of his condition. After discharge, the patient was given short-term oral vitamin supplementation and actively treated for chronic gastritis, encouraged to eat a nutritious and easily digestible diet, and instructed to perform vestibular rehabilitation training.

## 28.2 Case Study

The patient was a young male with a subacute onset, and his condition showed a continuous progressive aggravation. The main symptoms were eye movement disorder and ataxia. During the hospitalization, there were no clear positive findings in laboratory tests and no infarcts or occupying lesions in several brain MRI examinations, nor were there any abnormal signals in the medial thalamus, papillae, or around the midbrain aqueduct. In combination with the patient's history of chronic gastritis and low food intake over the years, a vitamin B deficiency was considered to be the cause of the disease, and the initial diagnosis of Wernicke's encephalopathy was made. After treatment with vitamin supplementation, the patient's clinical symptoms gradually resolved.

## 28.3 Case Review

Wernicke's encephalopathy was first reported in 1881 by Carl Wernicke, a German neuropsychiatrist. It is a metabolic disease of the central nervous system caused by vitamin $B_1$ deficiency, which is most often seen in people who consume large amounts of alcohol over a long period of time. Other conditions that can cause impaired absorption or increased consumption of the vitamin can also cause this disease, such as gastrointestinal disorders, prolonged dietary restriction, prolonged fasting with parenteral nutrition, and patients with malignant tumors. The diagnosis of Wernicke's encephalopathy needs to meet any two of the following criteria and to exclude other diseases. (1) A history of malnutrition or alcohol consumption. (2) Disorders of mental consciousness. (3) Oculomotor disorders. (4) Ataxia. Brain MRI is of great value in the diagnosis of Wernicke's encephalopathy, with a diagnostic sensitivity of 53% and a specificity of 93%. Abnormal signals on MRI may be seen in midline structures such as the medial thalamus, the papillary bodies, the midbrain aqueduct, the third and fourth ventricles, and therefore brain MRI should be the first choice when the disease is suspected. The treatment of Wernicke's encephalopathy is mainly high-dose vitamin B1 supplementation. Patients with this disease generally have a good prognosis if they are promptly diagnosed and treated, and delayed treatment can result in a poor prognosis and can even lead to death, and its residual ataxia and other symptoms after treatment can be improved by vestibular rehabilitation.

## Bibliography

Akdal G, MacDougall HG, Chen L, et al. Selective impairment of horizontal vestibulo-ocular reflexes in acute Wernicke's encephalopathy. J Neurol Sci. 2016;365:167–8.

Okafor C, Nimmagadda M, Soin S, et al. Non-alcoholic Wernicke encephalopathy: great masquerader. BMJ Case Rep. 2018;11(1):e227731.

Welsh A, Rogers P, Clift F. Nonalcoholic Wernicke's encephalopathy. CJEM. 2016;18(4):309–12.

# Part III

# Other Vertigo Disorders

# 29 Orthostatic Hypotensive Dizziness

Liya Shi and Xueqiang Shen

## 29.1 Summary of Medical Records

Patient, male, 46 years old. Complaint: recurrent episodes of dizziness for 2 years. Present history: The patient was clearly diagnosed with hypertension 2 years ago and often experienced mild dizziness with a feeling of intoxication and unsteadiness in walking, which gradually worsened in the past 1 year and became obvious after activity, accompanied by a skewed walk. He had consulted several tertiary care hospitals, all of which considered the sequelae of cerebral infarction and hypertension and gave appropriate symptomatic treatment, but his condition did not improve significantly. In the past 2 months, the patient's episodes of dizziness had become more frequent. Upon detailed questioning of the medical history, each episode of dizziness was associated with activities after getting up and sitting. Past history: 10 years of diabetes mellitus, combined with diabetic nephropathy, diabetic peripheral neuropathy, diabetic retinopathy and bilateral vision loss, currently controlled by subcutaneous insulin injections; and 2 years of cerebral infarction. Past history of smoking for more than 20 years, has quit smoking for 4 years; history of alcohol consumption for more than 20 years, has quit drinking for 6 years. Vestibular function examination: negative positional test, normal bilateral horizontal semicircular canal function in caloric test, no abnormality in visual oculomotor function examination, and cervical vestibular evoked myogenic potential asymmetry ratio was 27%. Supine and standing blood pressure measurements: 149–169/99–106 mmHg in supine position and 110–126/79–83 mmHg in standing. The patient's episodic dizziness and other symptoms were considered to be caused by orthostatic hypotension, and further examinations for hypertension were performed: ALD 182 ng/L, D-Renin 2.3 μIU/mL, ARR 79.1 in the upright position; while ALD 116 ng/L, D-Renin 1.8 μIU/mL, ARR 64.4 in the supine position. A definitive diagnosis of orthostatic hypotension was made. The patient was given some medical treatments and recommendation of lifestyle modifications to prevent the development of upright hypotension to reduce the occurrence of his symptoms such as orthostatic dizziness.

## 29.2 Case Study

The patient was a 46-year-old middle-aged male who complained of recurrent episodes of dizziness for 2 years. The diagnosis of the patient was easily influenced by his past history and was diagnosed as having sequelae of cerebral

L. Shi
Institute of Vertigo, Electric Power Teaching Hospital, Capital Medical University, Beijing, China

X. Shen (✉)
Institute of Vertigo, Third Medical Center, PLA General Hospital, Beijing, China

© Scientific and Technical Documentation Press 2023
X. Shan, E. Wang (eds.), *Interpretation of Vertigo Cases*, Experts' Perspectives on Medical Advances, https://doi.org/10.1007/978-981-99-6995-1_29

infarction without early definitive diagnosis because of his poor general condition, previous history of chronic diseases such as cerebral infarction and diabetic complications, and no obvious positive signs at the outpatient visit. The patient was admitted to the hospital for further examination and diagnosis, and vestibular vertigo was first ruled out, and with further history taking, the patient's vertigo episodes were mostly in sitting, standing, and after head movement, and improved in the flat lying position. Blood pressure was measured with149–169/99–106 mmHg in the supine position and 110–126/79–83 mmHg in the standing position, and then the patient was definitively diagnosed as orthostatic hypotension. The treatment of orthostatic hypotension is mainly directed at the cause of the disease, avoiding factors that may cause orthostatic hypotension. The main drugs for the treatment of orthostatic hypotension are fludrocortisone and the alpha-adrenergic agonist such as midodrine, etc. However, in view of side effect of drug and individualized differences, it is recommended that for patients with orthostatic hypotension, prophylactic and etiological treatment should be the main focus, and drug therapy should be used when necessary. Prevention of orthostatic hypotension is mainly to remind patients to get up slowly after lying down for a long time, do some limb movements before standing, sitting up a few minutes after waking up, and then gradually transitioning to standing, which helps to promote venous blood flow back to the heart, raise blood pressure, and avoid the occurrence of orthostatic hypotension and symptoms of induced episodic vertigo.

## 29.3 Case Review

Although the rate of outpatient diagnosis of vertigo-related diseases has increased in clinical practice, it is still limited by the timeliness of physical examination of patients, so many patients with poor treatment results are admitted to the hospital for further detailed examination when necessary to avoid underdiagnosis and misdiagnosis of the underlying disease. In this case, the patient was diagnosed through careful examination after admission, and his episodes of dizziness were caused by orthostatic hypotension.

Orthostatic hypotension, also known as postural hypotension, is defined as a significant drop in blood pressure when standing up from lying to sitting or standing, or from sitting to standing, or presents during an upright tilt test, with a decrease in systolic blood pressure of ≥20 mmHg and/or diastolic blood pressure of ≥10 mmHg, or a systolic blood pressure of <90 mmHg within 3 min. Orthostatic hypotension is highly age-dependent, with epidemiological study findings showing a prevalence of 5–10% in the middle-aged population and up to 30% or more in older adults. Upright hypotension is also closely associated with many common chronic conditions, such as primary hypertension, congestive heart failure, diabetes mellitus, and Parkinson's disease. Upright hypotension is difficult to detect in hospitalized patients due to the use of medications, bed rest, etc. It can be argued that there is a delayed effect in such patients and this insidiousness increases the risk of cardiovascular events, including acute myocardial infarction, heart failure, stroke, etc. This patient was a middle-aged male with an obese body type, low activity level, histories of previous smoking, alcohol consumption, diabetes mellitus, and cerebral infarction as risk factors for the disease. The patient had a previous history of hypertension for 2 years and was using a triple combination of angiotensin II receptor antagonists, calcium antagonists and beta-blockers for blood pressure control, which was suboptimal and increased the risk of orthostatic hypotension. Orthostatic hypotension occurs for four main reasons. (1) Decreased effective circulating blood volume, such as absolute hypovolemia due to blood and fluid loss after trauma or inadequate blood volume due to redistribution of blood after the use of drugs such as angiotensin. (2) Reduced cardiovascular responsiveness, seen clinically mainly in elderly patients with reduced cardiac compliance and reduced vascular responsiveness to sympathetic excitation. (3) Autonomic nervous system dysfunction and damage to any part of the human pressure receptor reflex arc can lead to an inability of peripheral vascular tone to change in response to postural changes, resulting in orthostatic hypotension, such as in patients with diabetic peripheral neuropathy, lesions around the vasomotor center, and using certain central sedatives, antidepressants, etc. (4) Increased release and concentrations of diastolic factors such as 5-hydroxytryptamine, bradykinin and prostaglandins in the blood can cause peripheral vasodilation and result in orthostatic hypotension. Orthostatic hypotension is a recognized risk factor for falls, syncope, and cardiovascular events.

Orthostatic hypotension is also a major cause of the development of orthostatic dizziness/vertigo. In 2019, the Barany Society has published diagnostic criteria for hemodynamic orthostatic dizziness/vertigo.

The diagnostic criteria for definitive hemodynamic orthostatic dizziness/vertigo were as follows:

(A) ≥1 episodes of dizziness/vertigo or unsteadiness induced by rising (i.e., a change in body position from lying to sitting or standing, or from sitting to standing) or present during an upright position, which subsides when sitting or lying down.
(B) Orthostatic hypotension, postural tachycardia syndrome or syncope is recorded during the standing or upright tilt test (head-up tilt test).
(C) Exclusion of other diseases or disorders.

The diagnostic criteria for probable hemodynamic orthostatic dizziness/vertigo were as follows:

(A) ≥5 episodes of dizziness/vertigo or unsteadiness induced by rising (i.e., a change in body position from lying to sitting or standing, or from sitting to standing) or present during upright position, which subsides with sitting or lying down
(B) At least one of the following accompanying symptoms: (a) general weakness or fatigue; (b) difficulty thinking and concentrating; (c) blurred vision; (d) tachycardia or palpitations.
(C) Exclusion of other diseases or disorders.

The publication of the diagnostic criteria for hemodynamic orthostatic dizziness/vertigo will help clinicians in the recognition and treatment of orthostatic dizziness/vertigo and orthostatic hypotension.

## Bibliography

Choi JH, Seo JD, Kim MJ, et al. Vertigo and nystagmus in orthostatic hypotension. Eur J Neurol. 2015;22(4):648–55.

Kim HA, Bisdorff A, Bronstein AM, et al. Hemodynamic orthostatic dizziness/vertigo: diagnostic criteria. J Vestib Res. 2019;29(2–3):45–56.

Kim HA, Yi HA, Lee H. Recent advances in orthostatic hypotension presenting orthostatic dizziness or vertigo. Neurol Sci. 2015;36(11):1995–2002.

Low PA. Neurogenic orthostatic hypotension: pathophysiology and diagnosis. Am J Manag Care. 2015;21(13 Suppl):S248–57.

Shaw BH, Garland EM, Black BK, et al. Optimal diagnostic thresholds for diagnosis of orthostatic hypotension with a 'sit-to-stand test'. J Hypertension. 2017;35(5):1019–25.

# 30 Postural Orthostatic Tachycardia Syndrome in a Child with Episodic Vertigo as the Main Complaint

Qinghua Zhang

## 30.1 Summary of Medical Records

Patient, male, 13 years old. Complaint: Recurrent episodes of vertigo for more than 8 years. Present history: The child's parents complained that the child first developed sudden vertigo with no apparent cause 8 years ago, with a sense of self rotation, accompanied by palpitations, nausea, vomiting, fear of opening the eyes, photophobia, and phonophobia, aggravated by position change. There were no symptoms of tinnitus and hearing loss during the course of the illness, nor were there any headache, blackouts, diplopia, facial palsy, dysfluency in speech, or disturbance of consciousness, and the child was not treated. Since then, the child had occasional dizziness and discomfort, which lasted for a short time and did not affect his normal study and life. In the past 10 months, the child had recurrent episodes of vertigo, mostly after strenuous exercise, with a feeling of spinning and weakness of the limbs, accompanied by palpitations, shortness of breath, nausea, and vomiting, without ear symptoms such as tinnitus and hearing loss. The vertigo attack usually lasted for several hours, and relieved after rest, especially after sleep. He had repeatedly visited several local hospitals, and ECG, cardiac ultrasound, EEG, brain MRI, and other examinations did not reveal any significant abnormalities. Since the onset of the disease, the child's spirit, diet, and sleep were fine, his urine and stool were normal, and his weight did not change abnormally. Past history: The child had a history of motion sickness; he had a history of head trauma in 2006, when he fell from a height and sustained a contusion to his head with two stitches, but no other abnormalities. Admission examination: general and otologic examination was unremarkable. No abnormal findings on audiological examination. Vestibular function examination: negative spontaneous nystagmus; negative positional test; caloric test showed normal bilateral horizontal semicircular canal functions; rotation test showed bilaterally symmetrical horizontal post-rotational nystagmus triggered by suddenly stopping after sustained rotation. The brain MRI did not show any significant abnormalities. Upright test: the child's heart rate was 92 beats/min in sitting position, and increased to 136 beats/min after 6 min of uprightness, with palpitations, shortness of breath, dizziness, and other discomforts. The ambulatory electrocardiogram suggested a minimum heart rate of 58 beats/min and a maximum heart rate of 159 beats/min. Based on the child's history, symptoms, and ancillary findings, a diagnosis of orthostatic vertigo due to postural orthostatic tachycardia syndrome (POTS) was made. During hospitalization, the child was treated with supportive and symptomatic treatments, including the methods to

Q. Zhang (✉)
Institute of Vertigo, Third Medical Center, PLA General Hospital, Beijing, China

© Scientific and Technical Documentation Press 2023
X. Shan, E. Wang (eds.), *Interpretation of Vertigo Cases*, Experts' Perspectives on Medical Advances, https://doi.org/10.1007/978-981-99-6995-1_30

increase the amount of salt in the child's diet and the frequency of water intake to increase the child's blood volume. The child was instructed to avoid sudden changes in position, prolonged standing and lying on the back, straining to defecate or urinate, hyperventilation, hot environments, overexertion, overeating, insufficient water intake, infection, and avoidance of carbonated beverages to avoid triggering or aggravating vertigo symptoms. After treatment, the child had fewer vertigo attacks and less vertigo than before.

## 30.2 Case Study

The patient was a 13-year-old boy with a history of recurrent vertigo attacks for many years. A positive postural test on electrocardiogram and an upright test showed a heart rate of 92 beats/min in the sitting position, which increased to 136 beats/min after 6 min of uprightness, with symptoms of palpitations, shortness of breath, and dizziness, which led to the diagnosis of orthostatic vertigo due to POTS. This is a rare clinical case of childhood POTS with vertigo as the first symptom. The diagnosis of POTS in children requires that all three of the following criteria be met simultaneously. (1) Manifestations of upright intolerance such as dizziness or vertigo, syncope, chest tightness, nausea, palpitations, headache, blurred vision, hand tremors, and cold sweats after uprightness. (2) A positive uprightness test and/or head-up tilt test (HUTT). (3) Other than other underlying diseases that can cause autonomic nervous system symptoms. Among the criteria for a positive HUTT is an increase in heart rate of ≥40 beats/min or a maximum heart rate of ≥120 beats/min in a child who is upright for 10 min, along with upright intolerance symptoms such as dizziness or vertigo, chest tightness, headache, palpitations, facial changes, blurred vision, lethargy, and even syncope after uprightness. It has been proposed that the observation time for HUTT heart rate in children can be shortened to 5 min, i.e., an increase in heart rate of ≥40 beats/min in 5 min; or a maximum heart rate of ≥130 beats/min (age ≤ 13 years) or ≥120 beats/min (age ≥ 14 years) in 5 min, meeting one of these criteria, the diagnosis of POTS is established. The pathogenesis of POTS is not well understood and may be associated with altered blood volume, autonomic dysfunction, abnormal Bezold-Jarisch reflex mechanism, muscle pump dysfunction, abnormal vascular endothelial function, viral infection, and mutations in norepinephrine transporter protein. POTS is treated with supportive and symptomatic therapy, including lifestyle modifications, salt supplementation, and increasing the frequency of water intake. When general treatment is ineffective, low-dose beta-blockers may be used. Small doses of beta-blockers and salt supplementation have been reported to be the most effective treatment for POTS.

## 30.3 Case Review

Childhood vertigo is most often seen in children with recurrent vertigo of childhood, benign paroxysmal positional vertigo, and motion sickness, whereas vertigo due to POTS in children is clinically rare and such cases are easily missed and misdiagnosed. POTS in children is a form of sinus tachycardia associated with postural changes and is most often seen in school-age children. The clinical presentation is an increase in heart rate of ≥40 beats/min or a maximum heart rate of ≥120 beats/min in 10 min when the patient is shifted from a lying to an upright position, with symptoms such as dizziness, headache, chest tightness, chest pain, pallor, long breaths, fatigue, exercise intolerance, aura syncope, and syncope without a significant drop in blood pressure. It is needed to exclude organic heart disease, upright hypotension, and vasovagal syncope, etc. The child had vertigo as the main symptom, and his vertigo episodes were associated with postural changes and vigorous activity, and occurred during the school age, which could easily be misdiagnosed as recurrent vertigo of childhood, benign paroxysmal positional vertigo, and motion sickness. In this case, the child presented with vertigo attacks induced by upright position, with symptoms of palpitations, shortness of breath, nausea, and limb weakness, etc. The vestibular function test showed negative for positional test, while the electrocardiogram showed positive for upright test, in which his heart rate was 92 beats/min in the sitting position and increased to 136 beats/min after 6 min of uprightness, so the diagnosis of POTS was clear. And POTS is also a major cause of orthostatic dizziness/vertigo. In 2019, Barany Society published the diagnostic criteria for hemodynamic orthostatic dizziness/vertigo and this case fulfilled the diagnostic criteria. This case also suggests that detailed history taking and bedside physical examination are required for the diagnosis of pediatric patients with vertigo, and diagnostic thinking should be comprehensive to avoid misdiagnosis and missed diagnoses.

## Bibliography

Arnold AC, Ng J, Raj SR. Postural tachycardia syndrome—diagnosis, physiology, and prognosis. Auton Neurosci. 2018;215:3–11.

Fedorowski A. Postural orthostatic tachycardia syndrome: clinical presentation, aetiology and management. J Intern Med. 2019;285(4):352–66.

Kim HA, Bisdorff A, Bronstein AM, et al. Hemodynamic orthostatic dizziness/vertigo: diagnostic criteria. J Vestib Res. 2019;29(2–3):45–56.

Sheldon RS, Grubb BP 2nd, Olshansky B, et al. 2015 Heart Rhythm Society expert consensus statement on the diagnosis and treatment of postural tachycardia syndrome, inappropriate sinus tachycardia, and vasovagal syncope. Heart Rhythm. 2015;12(6):e41–63.

# Swallowing Syncope

# 31

Jing Dai and Xizheng Shan

## 31.1 Summary of Medical Records

Patient, male, 69 years old. Complaint: Recurrent syncope for 2 years. Present history: The patient had a sudden onset of dysphagia during a morning meal in March 2016, followed by general weakness and confusion, which lasted for several seconds and then improved on its own. Since then there have been three or four episodes of the above symptoms, all of which occurred in the morning while eating. There was no blackout, diplopia, palpitation, chest tightness, dyspnea, headache, vertigo, limited limb movement, convulsions, or incontinence at each attack. Since the onset of the disease, he was normal in mental state, dietary and sleep, and bowel movements and had no significant change in weight. Past history: He was diagnosed with coronary artery disease and underwent coronary stenting (1stent) in 2013 at another hospital, with no clear history of hypertension or diabetes mellitus. No history of smoking, but small amount of alcohol consumption. Currently, he was taking aspirin enteric tablets regularly at 100 mg once a day, with no history of other medications. On admission: heart rate of 70 beats/min, normal cardiac rhythm, no pathological murmur was heard in all valve auscultation areas. Otolaryngological and neurological examinations did not show any significant abnormalities. MRA: no significant abnormalities were found. Fiber-optic laryngoscopy showed chronic congestion of the pharyngeal mucosa and bilateral vocal cords, with no abnormal findings. Upper gastrointestinal imaging: swallowing function was coordinated, all segments of the esophagus were smooth, no niche shadow or filling defect was seen, showing chronic gastritis. Echocardiography: slightly enlarged left atrium, small amount of mitral regurgitation, slightly low cardiac function. Twenty-four-hour ambulatory blood pressure monitoring: average blood pressure 119/64 mmHg throughout the day, maximum 154/89 mmHg, average heart rate 71 beats/min. Twenty-four-hour ambulatory ECG monitoring: sinus rhythm, second degree type II atrioventricular block, R-R interval >2 s for 3 times, maximum 2.9 s, showing ST-T alterations. There were palpitation symptoms during monitoring, but no syncope occurred. The cardiology consultation suggested that coronary angiography should be reviewed, permanent pacemaker implantation should be performed if necessary, regular use of secondary prevention medications for coronary artery disease, and avoidance of beta-blockers. The patient and his family were fully informed of the patient's condition and further treatment recommendations. The patient was discharged from

J. Dai
Institute of Vertigo, Third Medical Center, PLA General Hospital, Beijing, China

X. Shan (✉)
Institute of Vertigo, Electric Power Teaching Hospital, Capital Medical University, Beijing, China

© Scientific and Technical Documentation Press 2023
X. Shan, E. Wang (eds.), *Interpretation of Vertigo Cases*, Experts' Perspectives on Medical Advances, https://doi.org/10.1007/978-981-99-6995-1_31

the hospital for observation and follow-up. Discharge diagnosis: swallowing syncope and arrhythmia.

## 31.2 Case Study

This case is a rare case of syncope in which the syncopal episode was induced by swallowing. There are many causes of syncope, so detailed history-taking and physical examination are important. The patient was seen in the vertigo clinic, where the attending physician focused on the patient's vertigo-related history, ruled out vertigo and pre-syncopal episodes, and finally confirmed the diagnosis of syncope. In the search for the cause of syncope, attention was focused on the following aspects, such as the patient's age, past medical history, precipitating factors, and signs and symptoms during the attack. In this case, the patient was an elderly male who presented with episodic syncope, which occurred in the morning while eating, independent of the nature of the food and the speed of swallowing. Each episode of syncope was characterized by sudden loss of consciousness without aura symptoms, lasting for a short period of time, about several seconds to tens of seconds, and recovering on its own. The patient had a previous history of coronary artery disease and coronary stent implantation. Based on these characteristics, the focus was on the possibility that the syncopal episode was a swallowing-induced neuroreflex syncope or a cardiogenic syncope. The patient underwent upper gastrointestinal tract imaging, Brain MRI and MRA, echocardiography, ambulatory electrocardiography, ambulatory blood pressure, and psychological assessment during hospitalization to rule out the possibility of syncope due to anatomical and functional abnormalities of the esophagus, cerebrovascular disease, and situational stress disorder. Only the electrocardiogram showed significant abnormalities, and the results of the ambulatory electrocardiogram monitoring showed the presence of second-degree type II atrioventricular block with three R-R intervals >2 s. A prolonged R-R interval, i.e., ventricular arrest, can lead to a significant decrease in cardiac output, resulting in blackouts or syncope due to insufficient blood supply to the cerebral circulation. During feeding and swallowing, mechanical stimulation of the tongue and throat, esophagus, and stomach can cause reflex slowing of the heart rate, convulsions, and even loss of consciousness by provocation of the vagus nerve, usually lasting 10–15 s. For this patient, considering his previous history of coronary stent implantation, he was advised to review coronary angiography, take regular secondary prevention medications for coronary artery disease, avoid beta-blockers, and perform permanent pacemaker implantation, if necessary, to eliminate or reduce future syncopal episodes.

## 31.3 Case Review

Syncope is a transient loss of consciousness due to transient whole-brain blood hypoperfusion, characterized by rapid onset, transient, self-limiting, and capable of complete recovery, and other non-syncopal losses of consciousness such as seizures, head trauma, or pseudosyncope need to be excluded in the process of diagnosis. Based on the etiology and pathophysiological classification of syncope and to facilitate clinical judgment of syncope, the Chinese Expert Consensus on the Diagnosis and Treatment of Syncope (2014 Update) classifies syncope into three categories: neurally mediated reflex syncope; orthostatic hypotensive syncope; and cardiogenic syncope. Among them, neurally mediated reflex syncope is the most common, including vasovagal syncope, such as syncope caused by emotional factors (fear, pain, etc.) or upright position; contextual syncope, such as syncope occurring after coughing, sneezing, gastrointestinal stimulation, urination, post-exercise, post-meal, etc.; carotid sinus syncope and atypical syncope. Common causes of cardiogenic syncope are arrhythmogenic and hemodynamic syncope. Arrhythmias may include bradycardia, supraventricular or ventricular tachycardia, drug-induced bradycardia and tachycardia caused by abnormal sinus node function, abnormal atrioventricular junctional zone function; or inherited arrhythmia syndromes, such as long Q-T interval syndrome, Brugada syndrome, short Q-T interval syndrome, and catecholamine-sensitive ventricular tachycardia; heart valve diseases, acute arrhythmias caused by organic cardiovascular diseases such as myocardial infarction or ischemia, obstructive cardiomyopathy, cardiac masses, pericardial diseases, or cardiac compressions.

In terms of the onset characteristics of this case, the patient's syncope was most likely neurally mediated reflex syncope, but the patient was an elderly male with a previous history of coronary artery disease and coronary stent implantation and recent complaints of occasional palpitation, so cardiogenic syncope must not be missed. Some patients with vasovagal syncope may themselves have severe functional or organic disease, such as esophageal stenosis, diffuse esophageal spasm, esophageal achalasia, inferior wall myocardial infarction, rheumatic heart disease, after coronary artery bypass grafting, high atrioventricular block, sinus bradycardia, and pathological sinus node syndrome, which are likely to be the true causes of the syncope. The pathogenesis of swallowing syncope is not well understood. It is generally believed that during swallowing, impulses descending along the motor branch of the glossopharyngeal nerve pass through abnormal conduction in the region of the jugular foramen, return to the brainstem via sensory fibers, enter the nucleus of the solitary tract and spread to the dorsal nucleus of the vagus nerve, causing vagal hyperexcitability and triggering arrhythmias, a drop in blood pressure, syncope, and other reactions. Nerve impulses can also cause syncope via the periglottic portion of the glossopharyngeal nerve via the carotid sinus nerve like carotid sinus allergy. Swallowing syncope episodes are not related to body position, but related to the nature of the food swallowed, such as swallowing hard, cold, or spicy foods that predispose to syncopal reactions, often without significant discomfort before or after the syncopal episode. In addition, some people with unstable autonomic functions may also experience swallowing syncope. The mechanism may be sympathetic excitation due to tension during swallowing, followed by parasympathetic excitation with bradycardia and peripheral vasodilation, resulting in relative hypotension. In addition, hyperventilation due to tension and fear aggravates peripheral vasodilation and cerebral vasoconstriction through hypocapnia and respiratory alkalosis, resulting in decreased cerebral blood flow and promoting syncope. Swallowing syncope can be caused by a single factor or as a result of the interaction of multiple factors.

Syncope is mostly transient and situation-specific, and due to the uncertainty of the timing of syncope episodes, the positive detection rate of routine tests is extremely low during the actual diagnosis, which often makes it difficult to obtain a satisfactory diagnosis. In March 2017, the American College of Cardiology (ACC), the American Heart Association(AHA), and the American Heart Rhythm Association(HRS) jointly published the Guidelines for the Diagnosis and Management of Syncope, which mentioned that attention should be paid to identifying the features of history associated with cardiogenic and non-cardiogenic syncope at the early stage of consultation, focusing on the assessment of risk factors, including short-term risk (emergency outcomes and prognosis within 30 days of syncope onset) and long-term risk (12-month follow-up). The risk factors were male, age > 60 years, ECG abnormalities, history of cardiac disease, hypotension, and previous or current heart failure, tumors, cerebrovascular disease, diabetes mellitus, and renal function abnormalities. The etiology of some syncope cases can be determined by history and characteristics of syncopal episodes. In the patients whose etiology cannot be determined need further investigations, such as carotid sinus massage, upright position evaluation, electrophysiological monitoring, echocardiography, exercise test, cardiac catheterization, psycho-psychological evaluation, and neurological assessment. The ambulatory ECG played a key role in the management of this case. Compared with ordinary conventional ECG, dynamic ECG can continuously record ECG signals for 24 or 48 h, which is easier to capture transient abnormal ECG changes and can improve the detection rate of transient arrhythmias. Esophageal electrophysiological examination is also of diagnostic value in patients with suspected bradycardia, bundle branch block, or tachycardia, and is a simple and effective diagnostic method. If sinus bradycardia and cardiac arrest appear on the ECG followed by focal abnormalities on the EEG, the patient's EEG abnormalities are secondary and can be differentiated from primary epilepsy.

The prevention and treatment of syncope is primarily to remove the cause, but when the cause is unclear or current treatment is ineffective, then one may choose education, recurrence prevention, or intervention to prevent sudden cardiac death should be selected according to risk factor stratification. Treatment principles: neurally mediated reflex syncope is mainly treated with non-pharmacological treatment, avoiding triggers, early identification of prodromal symptoms, and taking measures to terminate the attack; cardiogenic syncope, on the other hand, is mainly treated with its underlying disease, and patients at high risk of sudden cardiac death should be treated specifically, and radiofrequency ablation, pacemaker implantation, and surgical procedures are feasible for different causes. Surgery can be used for treatment of syncope if caused by esophageal disease. If syncope is induced by vagus nerve excitatory drugs, the drugs can be discontinued or reduced, and vagus nerve inhibitors such as atropine or heart rate increasing drugs such as epinephrine can also be applied.

## Bibliography

Birnie DH, Sauer WH, Bogun F, et al. HRS expert consensus statement on the diagnosis and management of arrhythmias associated with cardiac sarcoidosis. Heart Rhythm. 2014;11(7):1305–23.

Corrado D, Wichter T, Link MS, et al. Treatment of arrhythmogenic right ventricular cardiomyopathy/dysplasia: an international task force consensus statement. Circulation. 2015;132(5):441–53.

Islam Z, Warricker F, Shah BN. Swallow (deglutition) syncope. Postgrad Med J. 2016;92(1090):489–90.

Liu WL, Hu DY, Guo JH, et al. Chinese expert consensus on the diagnosis and treatment of syncope (2014 updated version). Chin J Intern Med. 2014;53(11):916–25.

Saitoh T, Satoh H, Makino K, et al. Swallow syncope. Acute Med Surg. 2014;2(2):145–6.

# Recurrent Vertigo Due to Paraneoplastic Syndrome

32

Yun Gao and Kefei Zheng

## 32.1 Summary of Medical Records

Patient, female, 59 years old. Complaint: Recurrent episodes of vertigo for more than 10 years, aggravated for 3 months. Present history: The patient had sudden onset of vertigo with no apparent cause 10 years ago, lasting about a few minutes, with nausea, vomiting, and photophobia. Since then, vertigo attacks have recurred, with 2 or 3 attacks per year. In October 2014, the patient developed a feeling of dizziness and unsteadiness in walking after a "common cold," which has lasted since. Past history: no history of tumor. She was admitted to the hospital on January 12, 2015 for further treatment. Physical examination: body temperature 35.8 °C, pulse 72 times/min, respiration 18 times/min, blood pressure 150/80 mmHg, clear consciousness, bilateral involuntary eye movement with clonus, no regularity, bilateral pupils equal size and round, normal reflex to light, normal muscle tone of spine and limbs, finger-nose test still stable and accurate, negative alternation test, positive Romberg test, bilateral knee tendon reflexes were normal and symmetrical, bilateral Babinski's sign was not elicited. Otologic examination: no abnormalities in the external auditory canal and tympanic membrane. Nystagmogram: showing spontaneous nystagmus; visual smooth pursuit test showed a type III curve; gaze test and static position test showed nystagmus in all directions; optokinetic test showed symmetrical optokinetic nystagmus bilaterally; and rotation test showed basically symmetrical bilateral post-rotational nystagmus triggered by suddenly stopping after sustained rotation. Brain MRI: multiple foci of cerebral ischemia under the frontoparietal cortex bilaterally. The results of blood, urine and stool routine examinations, biochemistry test, coagulation function test, and cancer screening were normal, and erythrocyte sedimentation rate 36 mm/h. After neurology consultation, the preliminary diagnosis was peripheral vestibular vertigo, and the patient received methylprednisolone hormone shock treatment and circulation improving drugs, and nerve-nourishing drugs for 1 week, but the patient's symptoms did not significantly improve, and the ocular clonus persisted and did not diminish. On January 15, 2015, chest CT showed nodules in the right breast. Breast ultrasound: mild hyperplasia in bilateral breasts and multiple nodules in the right breast. Mammogram: scattered gravel-like calcifications were seen in both breasts, and two irregular high-density nodules were seen in the outer lower quadrant of the right breast connected each other in a dumbbell shape with poorly smooth margins and a diameter of about 1.6 cm, suggesting right BI-RADS

Y. Gao · K. Zheng (✉)
Institute of Vertigo, Third Medical Center, PLA General Hospital, Beijing, China

© Scientific and Technical Documentation Press 2023

X. Shan, E. Wang (eds.), *Interpretation of Vertigo Cases*, Experts' Perspectives on Medical Advances, https://doi.org/10.1007/978-981-99-6995-1_32

grade IV and left BI-RADS grade II. The patient underwent ultrasound-guided aspiration biopsy for right breast hypoechoic solid nodules and then received total right mastectomy and sentinel lymph node dissection at an external hospital. Postoperative pathological diagnosis: right breast invasive ductal carcinoma (grade II). The patient was then clinically diagnosed with (1) right breast adenocarcinoma; and (2) paraneoplastic syndrome. Postoperative chemotherapy was given for four courses and the patient's dizziness and unsteadiness in walking gradually improved. Review on December 9, 2016 showed negative Romberg test. Vestibular function examination: negative spontaneous nystagmus; normal visual dysmetria test bilaterally; visual smooth pursuit test with type II curve; optokinetic test showing bilaterally symmetrical nystagmus with normal gain; negative gaze test; normal horizontal semicircular canal function bilaterally on caloric test; normal findings for balance function examinations.

## 32.2 Case Study

The patient was a middle-aged female with a history of recurrent vertigo for more than 10 years. The vertigo was spontaneous and lasted for several minutes, accompanied by tinnitus in the left ear, and tinnitus was aggravated at vertigo attack, accompanied by nausea, vomiting, and photophobia, but was not accompanied by significant hearing loss. The patient had no previous history of tumor. On admission, the patient was in good general condition, with no other abnormal findings except for opsoclonus and a positive Romberg test. The nystagmogram showed spontaneous nystagmus, opsoclonus was also seen in the gaze test and position test, and the visual smooth pursuit test showed type III curve, but the findings of optokinetic test and rotation test were not significantly abnormal. The brain MRI showed no abnormal findings except for multiple cerebral ischemic foci under the frontoparietal cortex bilaterally. The patient's history and symptoms of vertigo seemed to be like atypical Meniere disease, but the physical examination and nystagmogram did not match the characteristics of Meniere disease. The patient was diagnosed as having vestibular peripheral vertigo and was given methylprednisolone hormone shock therapy, circulation-improving drugs, and nerve-nourishing drugs for 1 week, but the patient's symptoms were not significantly relieved after treatment. Breast ultrasound showed mild hyperplasia in the bilateral breasts and multiple nodules in the right breast. Mammography showed scattered gravel-like calcifications in both breasts and two irregular high-density nodules connected in dumbbell shape in the outer lower quadrant of the right breast, with less smooth edges and a diameter of about 1.6 cm, suggesting a BI-RADS grade IV disease in the right breast and a BI-RADS grade II disease in the left breast. The patient then underwent ultrasound-guided aspiration biopsy for the hypoechoic solid nodules in the right breast and followed by total right mastectomy and sentinel lymph node dissection at another hospital. The postoperative pathological diagnosis was infiltrative ductal carcinoma of the right breast (grade II). The diagnosis of right breast cancer with paraneoplastic syndrome was confirmed at this point. The patient's vertigo and other symptoms were manifestations of the paraneoplastic syndrome. After four courses of postoperative adjuvant chemotherapy, the patient's dizziness and unsteady walking symptoms gradually improved. The vestibular function test showed that the opsoclonus disappeared, the visual smooth pursuit test showed previous abnormal type III curve turned to normal type II curve, and other vestibular functions also showed normal.

## 32.3 Case Review

Paraneoplastic syndrome is a group of clinical symptoms associated with malignant tumors. It is not caused by direct invasion of tissues or organs by the tumor, but a kind of remote effect of malignant tumors. Paraneoplastic syndrome is mainly seen in small cell lung cancer, breast cancer, ovarian cancer, and thymoma. Breast cancer is now one of the most common tumors in women. Based on the involved sites and the associated symptoms, paraneoplastic syndrome due to breast cancer may include the paraneoplastic opsoclonus myoclonus (POM) paraneoplastic cerebellar degeneration, paraneoplastic retinopathy, stiff-person syndrome, primary lateral sclerosis, acute necrotizing myopathy, sensorimotor neuropathy, and other types. The misdiagnosis rate of paraneoplastic breast cancer syndrome is high due to lack of awareness of this disease. Although the incidence of breast cancer paraneoplastic syndrome is much lower than that of tumor brain metastasis, the presence of this syndrome often contributes to the detection and diagnosis of the tumor. The patient is a middle-aged postmenopausal woman, and women in this age-group have a high incidence of female reproductive system and breast tumors. Her disease course was long, with a chronic insidious onset and progressive worsening of symptoms, without triggers such as drugs, nutritional metabolic disorders, or radiotherapy. Vestibular function examination showed persistent opsoclonus with irregular oscillations in a predominantly horizontal direction, suggesting central vertigo. Brain MRI showed multiple foci of cerebral ischemia under the frontoparietal cortex bilaterally, which was considered to be a diffuse neurological injury. The patient had breast cancer at the same time, and her symptoms such as opsoclonus and vertigo were considered to be due to breast cancer paraneoplastic syndrome. After appropriate treatment for the breast cancer, the patient's symptoms such as opsoclonus and vertigo disappeared. POM is one of the typical paraneoplastic syndromes of the nervous system. Opsoclonus myoclonus syndrome (OMS) is a syndrome of disorganized, rhythmic, rapid, and variable eye movements in both eyes, independent of the direction of gaze, and may be accompanied by rhythmic action myoclonus, which may involve the trunk, limbs, and head. In this case, the first symptom was vertigo, followed by unsteadiness in walking and then rapid, disorganized, and irregular nystagmus, which is consistent with OMS, the annual incidence of which is only 0.01/100,000 as reported by Aquilina et al. Two cases of OMS associated with breast cancer have been reported abroad, and only two cases of POM have been reported in China. Mayo et al. studied 21 patients with opsoclonus from 1990 to 2011, three of which were associated with underlying malignancy (two breast cancers and one small cell lung cancer). The exact pathogenesis of POM is not well understood. Adult POM usually occurs in female patients with breast or ovarian cancer associated with Ri antibodies. However, not all patients with paraneoplastic syndrome have detectable antibodies against neurons. Altaha et al. reviewed 31 cases of breast cancer-associated neurological paraneoplastic syndrome between 1993 and 2003 and only 36% of the patients were positive for antibodies to tumor nerves, while 32% were negative and another 16% were positive for unknown antibodies. The majority of antibody-associated central nervous system paraneoplastic syndromes were found to develop without a direct relationship with antibodies and in association with cytotoxic T lymphocyte responses. The pathological changes in patients with POM may include diffuse loss of pukenocytes in the cerebellum, loss of neurons in the inferior olivary nucleus, and also show perivascular inflammatory cell infiltrates, mainly monocytes, in the cerebellum, brainstem, and soft meninges. As a result, patients often have a combination of positive signs of cerebellum and brainstem and signs of meningitis. POM still lacks a definitive and effective treatment. Various types of immunotherapy, including steroids, immunoglobulins, cyclophosphamide, and rituximab, have been effective in the treatment of POM. Previous studies have shown that the application of adrenocorticotropic hormone (ACTH) or corticosteroid and resection of the primary tumor can improve the clinical symptoms, and the opsoclonus and other symptoms in more than half of the patients can disappear after treatment. The spontaneous remission of POM symptoms has also been reported, but it is very rare. The prognosis of POM is poor, and Fanous et al. showed that 5 out of 14 patients with early-stage tumors associated with POM died of POM.

## Bibliography

Aquilina A, Dingli N, Aquilina J. Postintervention acute opsoclonus myoclonus syndrome. BMJ Case Rep. 2017;2017:bcr2017219859.

Fanous I, Dillon P. Paraneoplastic neurological complications of breast cancer. Exp Hematol Oncol. 2016;5:29.

# Optic Neuromyelitis Optica Spectrum Disease with Dizziness as the Main Clinical Manifestation

33

Chunqiu Fan and Weiya Ma

## 33.1 Summary of Medical Records

Patient, female, 48 years old. Complaint: Postural dizziness with persistent hiccup for 1 year, persistent dizziness for 1 month, diplopia with right-sided facial numbness and weakness for 15 days, admitted to the hospital on October 19, 2018. Present history: The patient began to experience dizziness with no apparent cause about 1 year prior to admission, with nausea and vomiting; her dizziness related to position, occurring in the upright position and relieved in the recumbent position, and also with refractory hiccup symptoms, which affected her eating. The dizziness was further aggravated, with two episodes of transient loss of consciousness, both lasting 1–2 min, without convulsions or incontinence, and the lowest blood pressure measured at that time was 74/65 mmHg. After blood and cerebrospinal fluid tests, she was diagnosed with "posterior polar area syndrome, dry syndrome, Hashimoto's thyroiditis, and orthostatic hypotension" and was given glucocorticoid shock therapy (methylprednisolone sodium succinate 1000 mg daily for 5 days). The patient's symptoms improved and she was discharged from the hospital; after that the patient was treated with oral prednisone acetate (60 mg per dose, once daily, reduced by 5 mg every half month, and 5 mg every month after 3 months) and cyclophosphamide (500 mg per dose, once every 15 days, intramuscularly), and oral hydroxychloroquine sulfate (100 mg per dose, twice daily), and the patient felt no discomfort, and her daily work and life were normal. Two months ago, the patient stopped cyclophosphamide and hydroxychloroquine sulfate as prescribed by the doctor. However, 1 month ago, the patient had another episode of dizziness with no obvious cause, no sense of visual rotation, no nausea or vomiting, dizziness was not related to position change, no longer with hiccup symptoms, but was accompanied by unstable walking and a feeling of stepping on cotton; blood pressure measured outside the hospital 150/100 mmHg, oral antihypertensive medication, no significant change in symptoms. The patient's dizziness worsened 15 days ago, and she developed diplopia, with double vision when gazing to the left and right with right-sided obliquity of the mouth, weakness of right-sided eye closure and cheek puffing, as well as right-sided facial numbness and increased self-conscious right tinnitus, without limb numbness and weakness, and without speech disorder and choking cough. The brain MRI performed outside the hospital suggested "abnormal signal on the right side of the medulla oblongata and pons," and she was admitted to the hospital for

C. Fan
Department of Neurology, Xuanwu Hospital, Capital Medical University, Beijing, China

W. Ma (✉)
Institute of Vertigo, Third Medical Center, PLA General Hospital, Beijing, China

© Scientific and Technical Documentation Press 2023
X. Shan, E. Wang (eds.), *Interpretation of Vertigo Cases*, Experts' Perspectives on Medical Advances, https://doi.org/10.1007/978-981-99-6995-1_33

further diagnosis and treatment. Since the onset of the disease, the patient had a poor diet, slept well, and did not show any significant weight loss. Past history: 15 years of tinnitus on the right side. Family history: denied family history of hereditary diseases and similar diseases. Father died of myocardial infarction and mother is healthy. Physical examination: blood pressure 130/87 mmHg in the supine position, 130/87 mmHg in the standing position. No murmur was heard in the vascular auscultation area. Neurological examination: clear speech, normal higher cortical functions, bilateral pupils were equally round, with sensitive reflex to light, no nystagmus, both eyes were slightly inwardly retracted, and white sclera may be seen when abduction of both eyes, right facial hyperalgesia, right peripheral facial palsy, right ear hearing loss, the Weber test was right-sided, bone conduction was better than air conduction on the Rinne test, the tongue extension was right-sided, the right lingual muscle fibrillation was visible, the right soft palate elevation was weak, the uvula was left-sided, the right pharyngeal reflex was weak, the muscle strength and muscle tone of the limbs were normal, the depth and superficial sensation of the limbs were normal, the finger-nose test and the heel-knee-tibia test were stable, the Romberg sign was negative, the tendon reflexes of the limbs were symmetrically active, and no pathological reflexes were elicited. Auxiliary examinations: brain MRI with enhancement showed abnormal signals in the right pons and medulla oblongata, with no significant enhancement of the lesion (Fig. 33.1). Serum thyroglobulin antibodies >2439 IU/mL, microsomal antibodies >1013 IU/mL, negative anti-SSA and anti-SSB antibodies (weakly positive at the first hospitalization), and other immune-related tests were negative. Cerebrospinal fluid-related tests: normal cerebrospinal fluid pressure, routine and biochemistry showing normal, negative for aquaporin 4 antibody (AQP4-IgG), anti-myelin oligodendrocyte glycoprotein antibody (MOG-IgG) and oligoclonal band (OB), normal IgG 24-h synthesis rate (blood and cerebrospinal fluid), negative for cerebrospinal fluid self-immune brain antibody and paraneoplasm-related antibody. Carotid ultrasound: bilateral internal carotid artery plaques. Diagnosis: (1) Optic neuromyelitis optica spectrum disorder (NMOSD). (2) Hashimoto's thyroiditis. Treatment: After admission, the patient was treated with thromboxane to improve circulation, methylcobalamin and vitamin $B_{12}$ to nourish the nerves, heptaosaponin sodium to reduce edema, antiplatelet and lipid-lowering drugs to stabilize the plaque. After 3 days, the patient felt reduced numbness on the right side of the face and improved movement of the eyes bilaterally, and on examination, the right eye showed less sclera when abducted. However, on the ninth day of admission, the patient's eye movement abnormalities worsened, and both eyes were fixed horizontally, unable to gaze left and right, but able to gaze up and down. After glucocorticoid shock therapy with methylprednisolone of 1000 mg, the patient's condition gradually improved. On examination: clear speech, both eyes gazed to the left side, leftward horizontal nystagmus could be seen when both eyes gazing to the left, no nystagmus in other directions, facial sensory symmetry, right peripheral facial palsy, right tongue extension, right lingual muscle fibrillation, right soft palate elevation force was weak, leftward hanging of the uvula, right pharyngeal reflex was weak, muscle strength and muscle tone of the limbs were normal, deep and superficial sensation of the limbs was normal, finger-nose test and heel-knee-shin test were stable and accurate. Romberg's sign was negative. The tendon reflexes of the limbs were symmetrically active and no pathological reflexes were elicited. The patient was discharged from the hospital with controlled disease. After discharged, she was treated with oral drugs, including prednisone 60 mg once daily, reduced by 5 mg every month; calcium D, 1 tablet once daily; famotidine 20 mg twice daily; and tretinoin 1 g twice daily. Post-discharge follow-up and treatment: 3 months after discharge, the patient's symptoms were completely resolved, no positive signs were found on physical examination, and immunosuppressive therapy was added. Six months after discharge, the patient was treated with oral prednisone 10 mg and immunosuppressive drugs without symptoms.

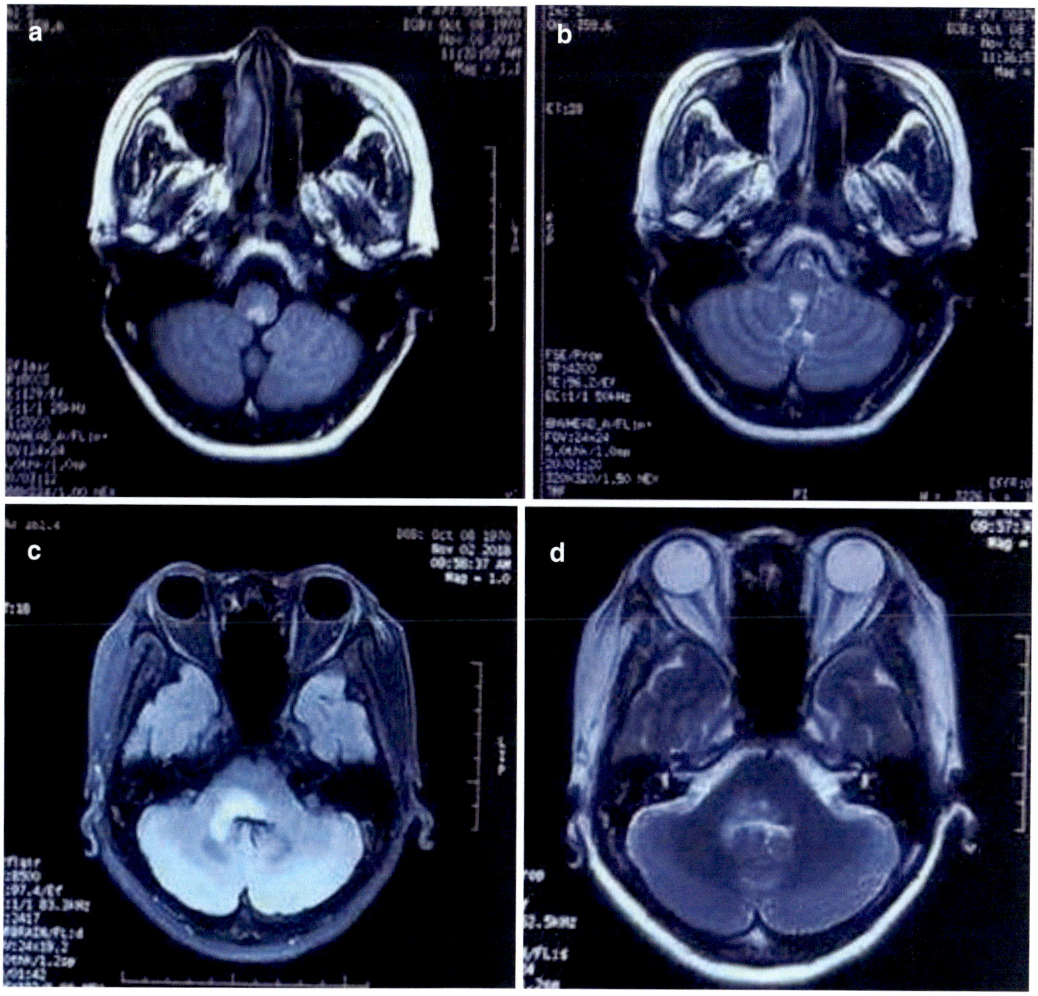


**Fig. 33.1** Brain MRI. Abnormal signal in the right pons and medulla oblongata with no significant enhancement of the lesion. (**a**) Medulla oblongata $T_2$ Flair; (**b**) Medulla oblongata $T_2$ WI; (**c**) Pons-oblongata junction $T_2$ Flair; (**d**) Pons $T_2$ WI

## 33.2 Case Study

The patient was a middle-aged female with two episodes of dizziness as the main clinical manifestation, the first with intractable hiccup, the second with double vision and right-sided facial numbness and weakness, the second admission to our hospital for further examination. The lesions were localized in the right vestibular nucleus, facial nucleus, trigeminal spinal tract nucleus, and right suspensory nucleus, and the brain MRI revealed right pons and medulla oblongata lesions. Cerebrospinal fluid examination was unremarkable, including negative AQP4. Application of hormonal therapy was effective. With comprehensive analysis, the diagnosis of NMOSD (AQP4-negative NMOSD) was made. International diagnostic criteria and Chinese guidelines state that the key to the diagnosis of NMOSD is a positive serum aquaporin-4 antibody (AQP4-IgG) and six core clinical symptoms. The diagnosis of NMOSD can be established even if the AQP4-IgG is negative and the lesion does not involve the optic nerve and spinal cord. Six core clinical symptoms include optic neuritis, longitudinally extensive transverse myelitis, area postrema syndrome, acute brainstem syndrome, acute mesencephalic syndrome, and acute cerebral syndrome. The patient had a remitting relapse and two episodes of lesions involving the area postrema and brainstem, which fulfilled the additional condition of MRI lesions, and therefore the patient was diagnosed as NMOSD (AQP4 negative).

## 33.3 Case Review

Two difficulties remain in the diagnosis of this patient.

1. How to diagnose NMOSD in the case of negative AQP4? Both international and Chinese guidelines proposed diagnostic criteria for NMOSD in the case of negative AQP4: the patient must have at least two core symptoms, at least one of which is optic neuritis, longitudinally extensive transverse myelitis, or area postrema syndrome, with spatial multiplex characteristics. Additional MRI conditions were met. The patient presented with a first episode of area postrema syndrome (MRI showed the lesion in the area postrema) and a second episode of acute brainstem syndrome (MRI showed the lesion in the right pons), so the patient had two core symptoms with spatially multiple features, the additional MRI conditions were also met, and thus the diagnosis of NMOSD was established.
2. How is NMOSD, combined with other immune system disorders, analyzed? The patient had been diagnosed with Sjogren's syndrome 1 year earlier (positive for SSA antibodies and SSB antibodies), and blood thyroglobulin antibodies >2439 IU/mL and microsomal antibodies >1013 IU/mL, indicating the presence of three immune-related diseases, including NMOSD, Hashimoto's thyroiditis, and Sjogren's syndrome. The guidelines stated that NMOSD is often comorbid with autoimmune diseases, including systemic lupus erythematosus, Sjogren's syndrome, and Hashimoto's thyroiditis.

After the diagnosis was made, the patient was treated according to the current treatment guidelines. After glucocorticoid shock treatment in the acute phase, the patient was given small doses of hormones and immunosuppressive drugs for long-term maintenance. The results of treatments and follow-up showed that the patient's symptoms were completely resolved at 3 months after discharge, with no positive signs on physical examination and additional immunosuppressive therapy; at 6 months after discharge, the patient was treated with oral prednisone 10 mg and immunosuppressive therapy, and no symptoms appeared.

## Bibliography

Kim HJ, Paul F, Lana-Peixoto MA, et al. MRI characteristics of neuromyelitis optica spectrum disorder: an international update. Neurology. 2015;84(11):1165–73.

Neuroimmunology Branch of the Chinese Society of Immunology, Neuroimmunology Group of the Neurology Branch of the Chinese Medical Association, Neuroimmunology Specialty Committee of the Neurology Branch of the Chinese Medical Association. Guidelines for diagnosis and treatment of optic neuromyelitis optica spectrum diseases in China. Chin J Neuroimmunol Neurol. 2016;23(3):155–66.

Wingerchuk DM, Banwell B, Bennett JL, et al. International consensus diagnostic criteria for neuromyelitis optica spectrum disorder. Neurology. 2015;85(2):177–89.

Zhang X, Li X, Deng B, et al. Analysis and comparison of clinical manifestations of patients with positive and negative hydantoin 4 antibodies in optic neuromyelitis optica spectrum disease. J Clin Intern Med. 2016;33(8):521–4.

# Acute Medullary Infarction Secondary to Hunt Syndrome

34

Jian Li

## 34.1 Summary of Medical Records

Patient, male, 41 years old. Complaint: dizziness and ear pain for 1 week. Present history: 1 week ago, the patient developed dizziness without any obvious cause, with a feeling of heavy head and light feet, no sense of rotation of vision, no symptoms of nausea or vomiting, tinnitus, ear fullness or obvious hearing loss. The patient was then admitted to the hospital for further diagnosis and treatment on March 19, 2018. Since the onset of the illness, the patient had no symptoms such as impaired consciousness, blackness in front of the eyes, speech impairment, difficulty in swallowing, choking and coughing, impaired movement of the limbs, and decreased visual acuity. Prior to admission, he had been diagnosed with herpes zoster in the right ear at an outside hospital and was treated with dexamethasone and other medications, with slight relief of ear pain and headache. Past history: There was no clear history of cardiovascular or cerebrovascular disease. Examination on admission: leftward horizontal spontaneous nystagmus was seen. Scattered herpes and crusts were seen in the auricular cavity of the right ear and the posterior wall of the external auditory canal, and the relaxed part of the tympanic membrane was congested. The external auditory canal and tympanic membrane of the left ear were not abnormal. The patient showed right-sided peripheral facial palsy: loss of right frontal lines, impaired eyebrow lift, incomplete eyelid closure, shallow nasolabial folds, leftward deviation of the angle of the mouth when showing teeth, normal soft palate lift, and no tongue extension deviation. Pure tone audiometry: sensorineural hearing loss in the right ear with a mean hearing threshold of 37.5 dB, predominantly high frequency hearing loss; normal hearing in the left ear. The tympanogram showed a normal "A" curve in both ears. Auditory brainstem evoked potential test: right ear response threshold was 30 dBHL, with slight delay in waves I-V and fair differentiation in all waves; left ear response threshold was 40 dBHL, with good differentiation in all waves and no delay in waves I-V. Vestibular function examination: positive spontaneous nystagmus with leftward horizontal nystagmus, maximum slow phase velocity 8.1°/s. Dix-Halllpike test and roll test were negative. Velocity step test: showing asymmetric slow phase velocity of post-rotational nystagmus for horizontal semicircular canals on both sides, significantly diminished on the right side. Caloric test: hypofunction in the right semicircular canal, with canal paralysis (CP = 84%). Posturography: anterior-posterior type instability with static eyes open or closed; sponge pad open eyes with a central pattern and sponge pad closed eyes with a diffuse shift. Brain MRI: no significant abnormalities were seen. Vestibular evoked myo-

J. Li (✉)
Institute of Vertigo, Third Medical Center, PLA General Hospital, Beijing, China

© Scientific and Technical Documentation Press 2023

X. Shan, E. Wang (eds.), *Interpretation of Vertigo Cases*, Experts' Perspectives on Medical Advances, https://doi.org/10.1007/978-981-99-6995-1_34

genic potentials (VEMP): diminished response on the right side. Based on the patient's history and ancillary tests, the initial diagnosis was Hunt syndrome. After admission, the patient was treated with drugs for antiviral, glucocorticoid, microcirculation improvement and nerve nutrition. After10 days, the patient's right ear herpes and facial palsy symptoms were less severe than before. But at 2 weeks after hospitalization, the patient felt dizzy worsening with nausea. Examination: torsional spontaneous nystagmus was seen. Repeated brain MRI: the right side of the medulla oblongata showed a point-like abnormal signal, suggesting acute lacunar infarction. CTA of the head: the right basal ganglia region showed infarct foci. The patient was treated with edaravone (30 mg each time, twice daily) and butalbital sodium chloride (25 mg each time, twice daily). After 1 week of treatment, the patient's symptoms improved, facial palsy was significantly reduced, and the right eyelid could be closed. Re-examination: spontaneous nystagmus was still seen, but showing leftward horizontal nystagmus. Brain MRI was repeated and it was shown that the punctate high signal on the right side of the medulla oblongata was reduced compared with the previous one, and thus lacunar infarction was considered. After continuing treatment for several days, the patient's symptoms of dizziness, headache, and otalgia subsided, and there was no longer any obvious manifestation of facial palsy, but hearing did not improve compared with before and spontaneous nystagmus was still positive for leftward horizontal nystagmus with a maximum slow phase velocity of 2.2°/s. The patient was discharged. He returned to the hospital 1 month after discharge for a follow-up examination, with no complaints of vertigo or dizziness, no manifestations of facial palsy, no positive localization signs on neurological examination, negative spontaneous nystagmus, and hearing as before.

## 34.2 Case Study

The patient presented with dizziness as the first symptom, followed by right-sided otalgia and ear herpes, and then right-sided peripheral facial palsy. Pure tone audiometry showed sensorineural deafness in the right ear with a mean hearing threshold of 37.5 dBHL, with predominantly high-frequency hearing loss. Vestibular function tests showed positive spontaneous nystagmus with leftward horizontal nystagmus, and velocity step test showed asymmetric slow-phase velocity of post-rotational nystagmus by suddenly stopping after sustained rotation on both sides, which was significantly reduced on the right side. The caloric test also showed the reduced function of the right semicircular canal, with canal paralysis (CP = 84%). The diagnosis of Hunt syndrome (type III) was clear on admission and was treated appropriately. However, at 2 weeks of hospitalization, the patient's ear herpes and facial palsy manifestations were significantly less than before, but his dizziness worsened with nausea, and on examination, torsional spontaneous nystagmus was found, and the brain MRI was reviewed for a suspected central lesion, and a punctate abnormal signal was seen at the right medulla oblongata, suggesting the presence of acute lacunar infarction, and cranial CTA showed an infarct focus in the right basal ganglia region. The patient's symptoms improved with pharmacological treatment, and the spontaneous nystagmus changed to horizontal nystagmus, and a repeated brain MRI showed that the punctate high signal in the right medulla oblongata was significantly reduced. The acute medullary infarction that occurred during the patient's hospitalization was detected promptly and treated appropriately, with a better outcome and prognosis.

## 34.3 Case Review

In 1907, Ramsay Hunt first reported a group of cases with specific symptoms caused by varicella-zoster virus infection of the geniculate ganglion of the facial nerve, which later became known as Hunt syndrome or ear herpes zoster, which is mostly unilateral and presents mainly with severe pain in one ear with ear herpes, hearing loss, and balance disturbance. This disease is also known as geniculate ganglion syndrome because of the presence of ipsilateral peripheral facial palsy. Clinically, the syndrome can be divided into three types based on the clinical presentation: type I, which presents with ear herpes only; type II, which presents with ear herpes and peripheral facial palsy; and type III, which presents with ear herpes and peripheral facial palsy, with hearing loss and vestibular dysfunction. Patients usually present with prodromal symptoms of viral infection such as general malaise, low-grade fever, headache, and loss of appetite at the beginning of the disease; followed by ear pain, which is often severe; usually presenting with herpes in the ear conchal cavity, external auditory canal, or tympanic membrane; and also may present with peripheral facial palsy, which is incomplete at the beginning and can rapidly develop into complete facial palsy within a few days or 2–3 weeks, usually reaching its peak in 10–14 days. Herpes and facial palsy may appear at different times, with most patients having herpes first, and a few patients having facial palsy before herpes, and in some cases, the herpes and the facial palsy are separated by 1 week or more. In addition, patients often have tinnitus, sensorineural deafness, vertigo, and balance disorders. Individual patients may also have symptoms related to the damage to the V, VI, IX, X, D, and XII pairs of cranial nerves.

The patient's first symptom was dizziness at the beginning of the disease, and herpes zoster in the right ear with otalgia appeared on the next day, followed by symptoms of ipsilateral facial palsy 3 days later. After admission, the patient's dizziness and facial palsy symptoms improved significantly with antiviral, neurotrophic, and microcirculatory medications. However, at 2 weeks of hospitalization, the patient experienced an increase in dizziness, and examination revealed that his spontaneous nystagmus changed from horizontal nystagmus at the time of admission to torsional nystagmus, because this rotational nystagmus suggested central nystagmus, which was mostly caused by lesions at the pons-oblongata junction, pontine arm, midbrain, etc. Therefore, further emergency brain MRI was performed, and acute medullary cerebral infarction was detected, and the patient was promptly treated with anticoagulation and microcirculation improvement drugs. The patient's symptoms improved after treatment because the infarct was small and mild, and the spontaneous nystagmus changed to horizontal nystagmus, and the repeated brain MRI also indicated that the medullary infarct was significantly improved. The patient was re-examined 1 month after discharge, and both Hunt syndrome and acute medullary infarction of the patient were cured.

## Bibliography

Bharadwaj S, Moffat AC, Wood B, et al. Herpetic cranial polyneuritis mimicking brain stem infarction-an atypical presentation of Ramsay Hunt syndrome. BMJ Case Rep. 2016;2016:bcr2016215182.

Ortiz GA, Koch S, Forteza A, et al. Ramsay hunt syndrome followed by multifocal vasculopathy and posterior circulation strokes. Neurology. 2008;70(13):1049–51.

# 35 Desensitization Treatment of Motion Sickness

Hui Leng

## 35.1 Summary of Medical Records

Patient, female, 24 years old. Complaint: Recurrent motion sickness for many years. Present history: For many years, the patient has experienced motion sickness when riding in a car, with varying degrees of symptoms, including dizziness, nausea, vomiting, sweating, pallor, rapid heartbeat, etc. She still felt tired and uncomfortable for a short time after riding in a car, and her appetite decreased, but after a certain period of recovery, the above symptoms disappeared completely. The patient often needed to take oral anti-motion sickness medication before each ride to control the symptoms of motion sickness. The patient had no significant headache symptoms and no hearing loss or tinnitus or ear fullness symptoms, and she was seen on June 9, 2017 at the outpatient clinic for the proposed desensitization treatment of motion sickness. Past history: no history of migraine, Meniere disease, benign paroxysmal positional vertigo, or other ear disorders. No family history of hereditary disease. Examination: General condition was good, blood pressure 110/70 mmHg. Otological examination: no abnormality of external auditory canal and tympanic membrane. Pure tone audiometry: normal hearing curve in both ears. Spontaneous nystagmus was negative. Vestibular function tests such as caloric test, velocity step test, cervical and ocular vestibular-evoked myogenic potentials (cVEMP and oVEMP), video head impulse test (vHIT), subjective visual vertical (SVV) and static posturography were not significantly abnormal, and the responses were basically symmetrical on both sides. Motion sickness Graybiel score: 11 points. Diagnosis: Motion sickness. Treatment: The patient underwent a "stepwise exercise program for motion sickness." The exercises were carried out through the SRM-IV diagnosis & treatment system for vertigo, with one exercise session every 2 days, for a total of ten sessions. The specific exercise program was as follows: (1) Vertical semicircular canal function exercise: 120° rotation in the right posterior-left anterior semicircular canal plane, 3 times clockwise and 3 times counterclockwise; 120° rotation in the left posterior-right anterior semicircular canal plane, 3 times counterclockwise and 3 times clockwise. The above steps constituted one therapeutic maneuver, with an interval of 10 s between each step. A total of ten therapeutic maneuvers were performed, the first three maneuvers were slow operations, i.e., each maneuver took 4 s with an acceleration of 120°/s; the fourth to sixth maneuvers were medium operations, i.e., each maneuver took 3 s with an acceleration of 150°/s; the last four maneuvers were fast operations, i.e., each maneuver took 2 s with an acceleration of 180°/s. (2) Horizontal semicircular

H. Leng (✉)
Department of Otolaryngology, Affiliated Hospital of Liaoning Traditional Chinese Medicine University, Shenyang, China

© Scientific and Technical Documentation Press 2023
X. Shan, E. Wang (eds.), *Interpretation of Vertigo Cases*, Experts' Perspectives on Medical Advances, https://doi.org/10.1007/978-981-99-6995-1_35

canal functional exercise: 180° rotation in the horizontal semicircular canal plane, alternating between counterclockwise and clockwise, for a total of 8 times. The above steps constituted one therapeutic maneuver, with an interval of 10 s between each step. A total of ten treatment maneuvers were performed, with the first three maneuvers being slow operations, i.e., 5 s/maneuver with an acceleration of 140°/s; the fourth to sixth maneuvers being medium operations, i.e., 3 s/maneuver with an acceleration of 160°/s; and the last four maneuvers being fast operations, i.e., 2 s/maneuver with an acceleration of 180°/s. Follow-up of patients after receiving the stepwise exercise for motion sickness. The results showed no significant difference in their vestibular function test results between pre- and post-exercise, and their motion sickness Graybiel score decreased to five points. The patient reported a slight reduction in discomfort during car rides after the fifth exercise session, a significant reduction in discomfort during car rides after the seventh exercise session, and almost no discomfort during car rides after the tenth exercise session.

## 35.2 Case Study

Based on the patient's complaints and history and the features of her clinical presentation, the case met the diagnostic criteria for motion sickness. (1) Normal mental state before the transport ride. (2) While riding the transport, the patient exhibited motion sickness-like symptoms such as dizziness, drowsiness, fatigue, mental discomfort, increased salivation, decreased appetite, nausea, and vomiting. (3) After leaving the vehicle, the above motion sickness-like symptoms gradually resolved or disappeared. (4) A history of recurrent episodes of similar symptoms during previous transport rides. The patient's medical history was clear, and the appearances of dizziness and other symptoms were not related to the change of head position but to the car ride, and the attacks of dizziness and other symptoms were not accompanied by hearing loss, tinnitus, ear fullness, visual abnormalities, photophobia, phonophobia, and other symptoms. The findings of various vestibular functional tests were normal. Therefore other common vertiginous disorders, such as vestibular migraine, Meniere disease, benign paroxysmal positional vertigo, vestibular neuritis, and so on, should be excluded, and thus the case was diagnosed as motion sickness.

Currently, the treatment of motion sickness consists of two main approaches: pharmacotherapy and non-pharmacotherapy. Medications for the prevention and treatment of motion sickness mainly include anticholinergics, antihistamines, sympathomimetic drugs, etc. Medications are not only slow to work but also need to be administered before each car or boat ride, especially since they have varying degrees of adverse effects, such as drowsiness, dizziness, dry mouth, blurred vision, etc., thus greatly limiting their application. The main non-pharmacological means of preventing and treating motion sickness are vestibular exercises and adaptations, and despite the variety of methods, there is a lack of highly desirable exercise program. In this case, the patient's motion sickness was prevented and treated by the SRM-IV diagnosis and treatment system for vertigo, and after the exercises, the patient's mean motion sickness Graybiel score was reduced to five points, and the various motion sickness symptoms were significantly relieved when riding in a car, and even no longer occurred, which achieved a better efficacy for the prevention and treatment of motion sickness.

## 35.3 Case Review

Motion sickness is a syndrome in which dizziness, epigastric discomfort, nausea, vomiting, cold sweats, pallor, and other vestibular and autonomic symptoms are induced due to the exposure to inappropriate motion stimuli. Motion sickness has a high incidence and also called as car sickness, seasickness, airsickness, and space sickness according to the environment in which motion sickness occurs. Motion sickness brings much inconvenience to people when they travel by transportation. Although many researchers have conducted a lot of in-depth research on the pathogenesis of motion sickness, the underlying mechanism is still not very clear. At present, the main mechanisms concerning the occurrence of motion sickness include the theories of sensory conflict (including the theory of intra-vestibular sensory conflict), otolith asymmetry, humoral shift, and so on. The occurrence of motion sickness is not only directly related to the intensity of motor stimuli, but also closely related to the individual susceptibility to motion sickness. Susceptibility to motion sickness is mainly associated with factors such as vestibular function, genetic characteristics, gender, age, and psychological factors. Motion sickness susceptibility is also increased in patients with certain vestibular disorders such as vestibular migraine, Meniere disease, and benign paroxysmal positional vertigo. The patient's history and symptoms in this case were typical, allowing for a definitive diagnosis of motion sickness.

At present, the prevention and control methods of motion sickness mainly include both pharmacological and non-pharmacological ways. Although anti-motion sickness drugs are an effective means for control of motion sickness, almost all anti-motion sickness drugs have varying degrees of adverse effects and their application is therefore somewhat limited. Habituation and adaptation, on the other hand, are the main avenues of nonpharmacological control of motion sickness. Various exercise methods have been tried to prevent and treat motion sickness, but there is still a lack of ideal exercise methods, for example, the existing training methods are not simple enough and their efficacies do not last long enough. In this case, the patient adopted a new exercise method to prevent and treat her motion sickness through the SRM-IV diagnosis and treatment system for vertigo, and achieved a good efficacy for the prevention and treatment of motion sickness. This exercise method and its efficacy need to be further investigated and improved in clinical practice. Therefore, in the process of performing the above-mentioned habituation exercise, close attention should be paid to the patient's status so that the habituation exercise program can be adjusted in a timely manner, such as the speed and acceleration of stimulation can be appropriately changed to achieve the best habituation exercise efficacy. In addition to the traditional pharmacological and non-pharmacological prevention and treatment pathways, Chinese herbal medicine such as herbal soup, acupuncture, and massage points are also commonly used as a means of prevention and treatment of motion sickness. Therefore, if the above-mentioned exercise methods are not effective in the prevention and treatment of motion sickness, they can be combined with acupuncture treatment, such as taking Baihui, Sishencong, Neiguan, Feosanli, and Hegu points. Modern research has shown that acupuncture has the effects of relaxing the cerebral cortex and inducing a sense of comfort, and acupuncture can promote sympathetic and parasympathetic synaptic connections and agitate the central nervous system, which helps to inhibit the occurrence of motion sickness.

## Bibliography

Golding JF. Motion sickness. Handb Clin Neurol. 2016;137:371–90.

Previc FH. Intravestibular balance and motion sickness. Aerosp Med Hum Perform. 2018;89(2):130–40.

Schmäl F. Neuronal mechanisms and the treatment of motion sickness. Pharmacology. 2013;91(3–4):229–41.

Shan X, Peng X, Wang E, et al. Preliminary observation on the effect of high-intensity vestibular function exercise to prevent and treat motion sickness. Beijing Med. 2017;39(1):1–5.

Strupp M, Brandt T, Huppert D, et al. Prevalence of motion sickness in various vestibular disorders: a study on 749 patients. J Neurol. 2018;265(Suppl 1):95–7.

MIX
Papier aus verantwortungsvollen Quellen
Paper from responsible sources
FSC® C105338

If you have any concerns about our products,
you can contact us on
**ProductSafety@springernature.com**

In case Publisher is established outside the EU,
the EU authorized representative is:
**Springer Nature Customer Service Center GmbH**
**Europaplatz 3, 69115 Heidelberg, Germany**

Printed by Libri Plureos GmbH
in Hamburg, Germany